Suprachoroidal Space Interventions

Shohista Saidkasimova • Thomas H. Williamson

Editors

Suprachoroidal Space Interventions

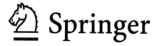 Springer

Editors
Shohista Saidkasimova
Tennent Institute of Ophthalmology
Glasgow, UK

Thomas H. Williamson
Department of Ophthalmology
St. Thomas' Hospital
London, UK

ISBN 978-3-030-76855-3   ISBN 978-3-030-76853-9   (eBook)
https://doi.org/10.1007/978-3-030-76853-9

This Springer imprint is published by the registered company Springer Nature Switzerland AG
The registered company address is: Gewerbestrasse 11, 6330 Cham, Switzerland

Contents

Anatomy and Physiology of the Suprachoroidal Space

Shohista Saidkasimova

Introduction

The suprachoroid is located between the sclera and choroid, stretching from the ciliary body to the optic nerve. Historically the suprachoroidal space (SCS) was often described in association with severe complications such as suprachoroidal haemorrhage and choroidal effusions. More recently, we have rediscovered the space for its potential for aqueous outflow, drug delivery, surgical treatment of retinal detachment, and an access route for the delivery of the gene therapy, stem cells and retinal implants. Advances in imaging have significantly increased our ability to visualise the choroid and suprachoroidal space in vivo, providing a better opportunity to study their relationship in health and disease.

A thorough understanding of the anatomy and physiology of the suprachoroidal space will help to maximise the benefits and minimise the risk of complications associated with this approach. The anatomical and physiological studies of the suprachoroidal space are technically challenging and are more often performed on animals. We tried to focus on human and primate studies in our descriptions, bearing distinctive differences between species, i.e. in choroidal and lymphatic vasculature, focusing function etc.

S. Saidkasimova (✉)
Tennent Institute of Ophthalmology, Glasgow, UK
e-mail: shohista@doctors.org.uk

© The Author(s), under exclusive license to Springer Nature Switzerland AG 2021
S. Saidkasimova, T. H. Williamson (eds.), *Suprachoroidal Space Interventions*,
https://doi.org/10.1007/978-3-030-76853-9_1

1

Embryogenesis

Formation of optic vesicles from the neuroectoderm and their evagination leads to the development of the optic cup. It's walls become precursors of the retina and the retinal pigment epithelium (RPE) [1–6]. Surrounding mesenchyme and neuroectoderm form the outer layers of the eyeball, including the choroid and sclera from the 7–8 week of gestation. The development of the suprachoroid takes place relatively late in the embryogenesis. Since the eye develops inside out, the sclera and therefore the suprachoroid are one of the later structures to form. The sclero-choroidal border is not identifiable at 7 weeks of gestation but starts to become visible at week 12 as the two layers of mesenchymal condensation surrounding the optic cup differentiate into the sclera and choroid, starting anteriorly and reaching posterior pole by week 13 [3]. The maturation of the choroid and suprachoroid continues into week 24 [2, 7], and accumulation of pigment continues throughout gestation [8].

Sclera

The outer layer of the eyeball, the sclera, provides a protective coat for its contents. It is approximately 1 mm thick, varying in thickness from 0.3–1.2 mm and covers >90% of the surface area of the eye [9].

The sclera is made of mainly collagen type 1 fibres of varying sizes, 62–125 nm [10]. It also has a large number of elastin fibres closer to the inner surface of the sclera facing the suprachoroidal space [11]. Collagen and elastin fibres are embedded in the extracellular matrix, made of proteoglycans and glycosaminoglycans [12]. The latter are able to bind large amounts of water [13] facilitating the trans-scleral hydraulic conductivity. Also, matrix metalloproteinase (MMP) enzymes, capable of degrading proteoglycans and collagen, are stored in an inactive form in the sclera and can be activated during inflammation and growth [14].

The scleral globe has a mean diameter of 24 mm; however, in highly myopic eyes, the eye's shape may change and form outpouchings, or staphylomata, with thinning of sclera, choroid and retina [14, 15].

The sclera forms the outer boundary of the suprachoroid and has several openings to allow vessels and nerves into the eye (Fig. 1). The largest opening in the sclera posteriorly is the scleral canal, which is 1.8 mm in diameter. The outer two-thirds of the scleral collagen merge with the optic nerve's dura mater (Fig. 2).

Choroid

The choroid is a highly vascular structure and forms the inner wall of the SCS. It has a high blood flow, that is necessary to support the high metabolic needs of the outer retina and photoreceptors [1]. The pigment contained within the choroid helps to

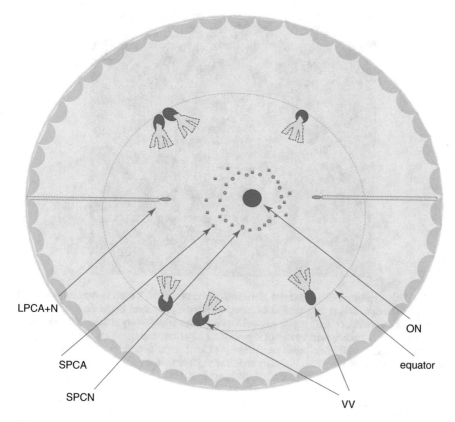

LPCA+N

SPCA

SPCN

ON

equator

VV

Fig. 1 The diagram of the internal surface of the scleral openings for the optic nerve (ON), short posterior ciliary nerves (SPCN), short posterior ciliary arteries (SPCA), long posterior ciliary arteries and nerves, lateral and medial (LPCA+N), and vortex veins (VV)

absorb the excess light and the heat [16], and it's intrinsic growth factors and enzymes (MMP) play a role in the development and growth of the choroid, and maintenance of its function [17–22].

The choroidal vascular network is supported by branches of short and long posterior ciliary arteries. The choroid is arranged in layers of vessels: the outer large vessel layer (Haller's), medium-sized vessel layer (Sattler's), and the choriocapillaris, an inner layer of fenestrated capillaries, although no distinct border between the layers exists [14]. Blood from the choroid is drained mainly via vortex veins posteriorly, but also the anterior ciliary veins anteriorly (Fig. 3).

Arterial and venous networks have a separate segmental organisation in the choroid with watershed zones between segments which are visible on an angiogram [14, 23]. The choroidal vessels are immersed in the connective tissue with pigment cells, smooth muscle cells [24, 25], and intrinsic neurons [26].

The choroid is attached to the sclera by strands of connective tissue, which are easily separated anteriorly opening the suprachoroidal space (SCS).

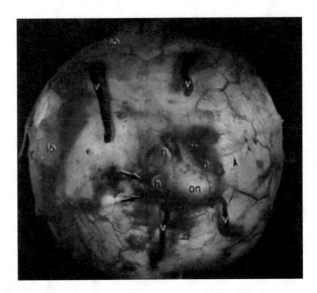

Fig. 2 The posterior surface of the eye globe shows vortex veins (*v*), optic nerve (on), muscular tendon of inferior oblique (*io*), tendon of superior oblique (*so*), short posterior ciliary arteries (*arrows*), short posterior ciliary nerves (*n*), and long posterior ciliary artery and nerve (*arrowhead*). A wreath of short posterior ciliary nerves is prominent superiorly and inferiorly. Temporal (*left* of optic nerve) and nasal (*right* of optic nerve) canals of long posterior arteries and nerves mark the horizontal meridian of the globe. Emissary canals of the four vortex veins lie in the oblique quadrants. (Reproduced with permission from R. Buggage et al, [1])

Suprachoroid

The suprachoroid (synonymous with lamina suprachoroidea, lamina fusca, suprachoroidea and suprachoroidal space) is a thin layer of approximately 10–34μm in height [27, 28] between the sclera and choroid. The most accurate term would be lamina suprachoroidea (or shorter suprachoroid) since it describes a layer of heterogenous connective tissue with embedded cells of mixed origin, distinct in structure from adjacent choroid and sclera, and there is no anatomical space as such in physiological conditions. The collagen fibres of the suprachoroid provide only loose attachment of the choroid to the sclera and act as a cleavage plane for separation surgically or in pathological conditions. Therefore, the SCS is not inappropriately referred to as a potential space. However, for convenience, we will interchangeably use the terms suprachoroid to describe anatomical structure in physiologic conditions and the SCS when describing pathologic changes or surgical interventions.

The suprachoroid is continuous over the circumference of the eye from the firm attachment of the ciliary body to the scleral spur anteriorly to the optic nerve posteriorly. It is referred to as the supraciliary space over the ciliary body and suprachoroidal space over the choroid. It is pinned by vessels and nerves traversing it, most prominently by vortex veins.

The early descriptions of suprachoroid and perichoroidal space were based on detailed studies by Gray [29, 30] and Salzman [31]. In macroscopic studies, they

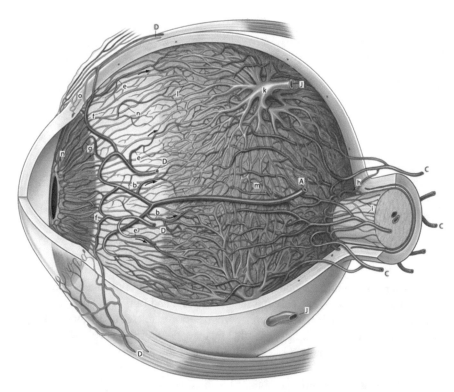

Fig. 3 The choroidal blood vessels. (*A*) Long posterior ciliary arteries, entering nasally and temporally along the horizontal meridian. These two arteries give off three to five branches (*b*) at the orra serrata to supply the anterior choriocapillaris. The short posterior ciliary arteries enter the choroid around the optic nerve (*c*). (*D*) Anterior ciliary arteries enter the eye through the rectus muscles and give off 8 to 12 branches (*e*) that pass back through the ciliary muscle to join the anterior choriocapillaris. The vortex veins exit from the eye through the posterior sclera (*J*) after forming an ampulla (*k*) near the internal sclera. The venous return from the iris and ciliary body (*n*) is mainly posterior into the vortex system, but some veins cross the anterior sclera and limbus (*o*) to enter the episcleral system of veins. (Reproduced with permission from Hogan MJ, 1971 [27])

described lamina fusca and lamina suprachoroidea as two separate structures following their iatrogenic separation in the ex vivo specimen into two parts attached to either sclera or choroid. In the histological specimens, such separation could not be identified [32, 33] (Fig. 4).

Traditional studies of the anatomy and physiology of the suprachoroid in human were mainly ex-vivo by dissection [29], light and electron microscopy of the histological slides [27, 32, 33], vascular resin casts [34–38], immunohistochemistry [24], and fluid dynamic studies [39–41]. Whilst ex-vivo studies may allow a description in great detail, the natural proportions of tissues (the vessels and SCS) can be distorted [36, 38]. In vivo ultrasound studies can identify the SCS in pathological conditions. The recent introduction of high-resolution enhanced depth OCT allowed visualisation of the suprachoroid in physiological conditions [42–44].

Fig. 4 Sclerochoroidal
junction cross section,
H&E stain (×100). *R*
retina, *Ch* choroid, *Su*
suprachoroid, *Sc* sclera.
(Courtesy of Dr. Fiona
Roberts, Glasgow UK)

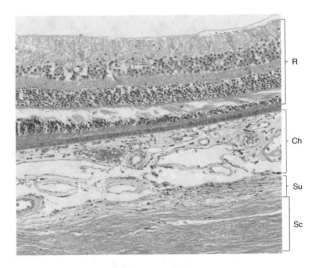

Cadaver corrosion cast studies of the SCS showed smooth outer surface and uneven inner surface with a vascular pattern (Krohn and Bertelsen, 1997b, 1997a). The hemispherical casts had a mean anteroposterior diameter of 13 mm and a circumferential width of 17 mm. The methyl methacrylate resin was able to stretch the SCS to up to 4 mm in height but remained thin at the points of traversing vessels crossing the cast [36].

The suprachoroid is darkly pigmented when accessed in vivo. The term "lamina fusca" (from Latin "black layer") was attributed to the pigment present in the suprachoroid. The distribution of the pigment is uneven, and the suprachoroid is more pigmented posteriorly than anteriorly. Also, the pigment thins over the nerves and vessels, sometimes with a darker demarcation line which makes them visible on fundoscopy, most prominently along the long posterior ciliary arteries and nerves at the horizontal 3 and 9 o'clock meridia. Similar landmarks exist along the vertical meridia, marked by ciliary arteries and nerves with a 15° tilt temporally in the superior and nasally in the inferior hemisphere [46] (Fig. 5).

Histological studies of the suprachoroid revealed tightly packed cells and fibres traversed by the vessels and nerves [27]. Their relationship becomes more apparent when separated by accumulated fluid in the pathologic conditions or post-mortem studies. Cells and structures in the suprachoroid can be divided into the following groups:

Collagen fibres form the bulk of the suprachoroid. Here they change from less orderly orientation around the choroidal vasculature to a more linear orientation almost parallel to the scleral fibres. They travel somewhat obliquely but almost

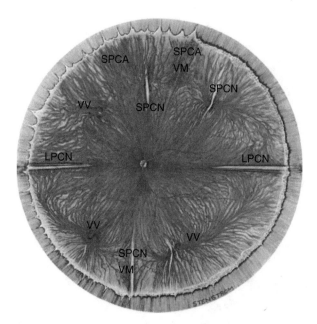

Fig. 5 Normal fundus appearance, left eye. *SPCA* short posterior ciliary arteries, *SPCN* short posterior ciliary nerves, *LPCN* long posterior ciliary nerves, *VV* vortex veins; (Modified with permission from Ruthin U, Schepens C, 1967. [53])

parallel to the sclera, starting from their attachment to the collagen fibres of the ciliary body and choroid anteriorly and intertwine with the scleral collagen posteriorly [31]. The fibres that start at the equator have a shorter and more oblique course. On dissection, the strings of collagen lamellae remain attached to the choroid giving it an uneven surface appearance. On the histological section 6–8 rows of collagen lamellae can be found [31]. The length of the collagen fibres does not strengthen the adhesion of the sclera to the choroid, especially anteriorly allowing easy separation. This may have physiological advantages for the suprachoroid to function as a buffer zone for a transudate, which can build up as a result of increased uveoscleral outflow, gradient pressure imbalance or increased venous outflow resistance, allowing diversion of the accumulated fluid away from the fovea, where fibres are shorter and fluid accumulates only in extreme pathological conditions.

Elastic fibres travel at an angle to the collagen fibres and help maintain the tight opposition of the sclera to the choroid in a healthy eye (Fig. 6). The elastic fibres are

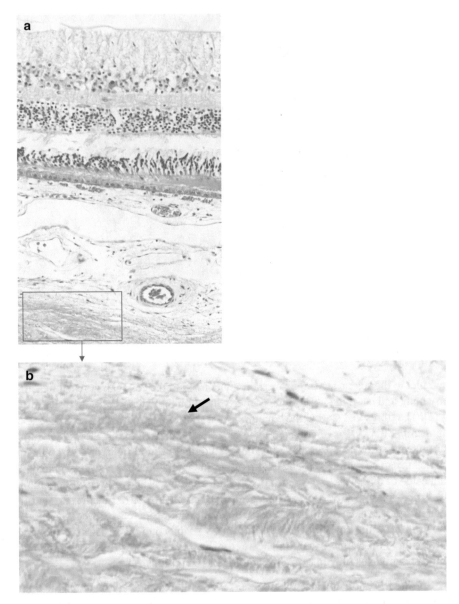

Fig. 6 (a) Sclerochoroidal junction cross section, H&E stain (×100). Suprachoroid cross-section stained with H&E stained section (×200). (b) Magnified view of section shown. Elastin fibres stained silvery grey (black arrow) (Courtesy of Dr. Fiona Roberts, Glasgow, UK)

denser in the posterior pole and less so anteriorly, explaining the more anterior distribution of choroidal effusion in a hypotonus eye.

Melanocytes are the most numerous cells in the SCS. They have a star shape with fenestrated processes which have been shown to intertwine with processes of fibroblastic cells in the macaque monkey [47]. Forming 5–10 layers, melanocytes are 20–30μm long and contain melanosomes [32, 48]. Melanocytes are most abundant in the layers adjacent to the choroid. However, they can also be seen in the loose collagen of the inner sclera (Fig. 7). Their distribution in the circumference of the eye is denser in the posterior pole compared to the anterior part, suggesting a possible role in visual function by the absorption of excess light. They are smaller than those in the choroidal stroma [49].

Fibroblasts are the second most numerous cells in the suprachoroid arranged in multiple layers interspersed with pigment cells. They have scarce cytoplasm and long processes with pore-like fenestrations; a reticular network is seen next to fibrocytes [27]. Gap junctions, intermediate junctions, and isolated tight junctions without zonulae occludens are present between the fibroblasts [32]. Fibroblasts are responsible for producing the collagen fibres [7] and the hyaluronate of the extracellular matrix.

Nonvascular smooth muscle cells (NVSMC) are found in abundance in the suprachoroid and adjacent choroid. They are most plentiful at the posterior pole and organised in an orderly fashion around the vessels and nerves [24, 50] (Fig. 8). May et al. described five groups of α-actin containing myocytes in the SCS: arcuate

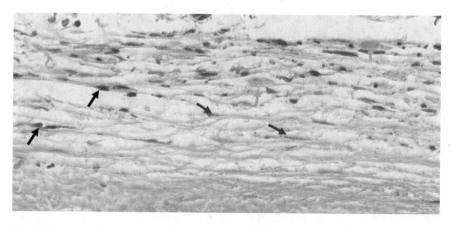

Fig. 7 The suprachoroid, H&E stained section (×200). Cells marked with arrows: Fibroblasts (purple arrow); Ganglion cells (green arrow); melanocytes (black arrow). (Courtesy of Dr. Fiona Roberts, Glasgow UK)

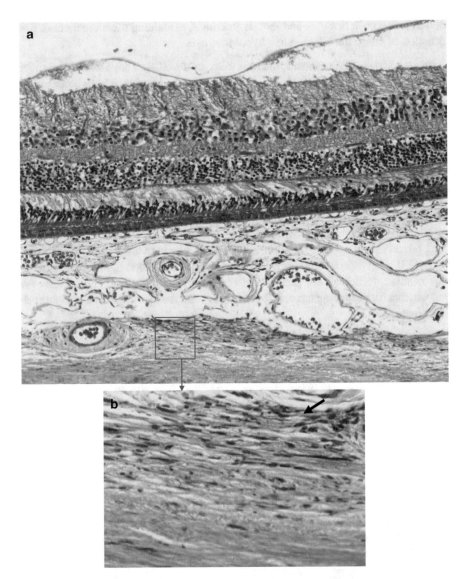

Fig. 8 Suprachoroid cross-section stained with Massons trichrome stain, ×40 (**a**). Smooth muscle cells stained red (black arrow) ×200 (**b**). (Courtesy of Dr. Fiona Roberts, Glasgow UK)

orientation around the exit points of the short and long posterior arteries, nerves and vortex veins; along the vessels in the outer choroid, and a separate group in the macular region of the SCS in adults but not in the newborns [24] (Fig. 9). They may play a role in regulating the blood flow, but the exact role is unknown. Hogan et al. had likened the vascular choroid to erectile tissue [27] due to its ability to change the thickness, in turn, partially attributed to the smooth muscle cells. The later

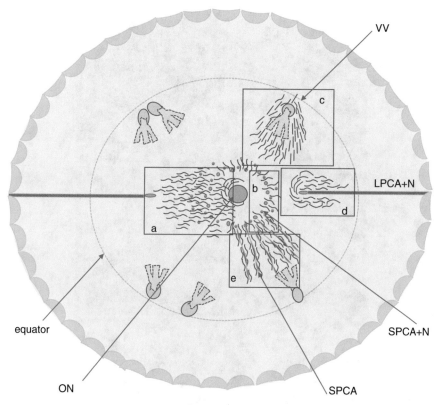

Fig. 9 Schematic drawing of the distribution of non-vascular smooth muscle cells in the suprachoroid, right eye (NVSMC; blue lines representing direction of cells): (**a**) plaque-like arrangement of NVSMC in the foveal region, spreading up to the temporal rim of the optic nerve; (**b**) around the entry points of short posterior ciliary arteries; (**c**) Around the vortex veins (VV); (**d**) around long posterior ciliary artery and nerve (LPCA+N); (**e**) along the short posterior ciliary arteries (SPCA) (Based on the findings of May et al., 2005 [24])

development and predominant position of NVSMC within the visual axis suggest a possible role in focusing via choroidal thickness adjustment.

Multipolar and bipolar ganglion cells are scattered in the suprachoroid (Fig. 10). They belong to the group of intrinsic choroidal neurons and their exact role is unknown.

Also seen in the suprachoroid are the migrating cells, including the macrophages, lymphocytes and occasional plasma cells.

Extracellular Matrix (ECM) The main components of the ECM are the collagen and elastic fibres, which are closely linked and are similar in composition to those of the sclera and the choroid, and glycosaminoglycans (aggrecan, biglycan, and decorin) which are shared with the sclera [10]. Another common glycosaminoglycan is the innate hyaluronic acid, produced by fibroblasts. Matrix

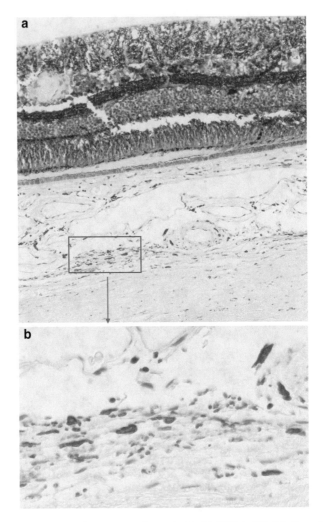

Fig. 10 Sclerochoroidal junction cross-section stained with NSE (x100) (**a**). Suprachoroid cross-section stained with NSE (x200) (**b**). Dendritic nerve cells are stained in brown colour. (Courtesy of Dr. Fiona Roberts, Glasgow UK)

metalloproteinases contribute to the ECM remodelling and regulation of the uveo-scleral outflow [51].

Vessels in the Suprachoroid

The suprachoroid has no innate capillary system. The vessels and nerves traversing it are destined for the choroid, ciliary body and iris (Fig. 11). Krohn & Bertelsen have shown two patterns of vascular passage in the suprachoroid of a human eye in

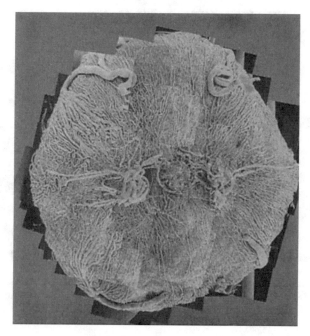

Fig. 11 Photomontage of the cast of the posterior pole of a right eye showing temporal and medial short posterior ciliary arterial bundles supplying choroidal vasculature and retrolaminar optic nerve vasculature. The lateral and medial long posterior ciliary arteries have been truncated at the equator. Vortex veins are clearly seen (Reproduced with permission from JM Olver, 1990;4 (2):262–72)

their methyl methacrylate casts: vessels that passed straight through the SCS and those which appeared to originate from the SCS itself before merging with a fine scleral venous capillary network. Additionally, their casts showed perivascular escape of the resin along the long anterior ciliary arteries and vortex veins [45].

The ophthalmic artery gives off lateral and medial branches of posterior ciliary arteries, each then divides into one long and numerous short posterior ciliary arteries.

Short Posterior Ciliary Arteries (SPCA) Approximately 15–20 branches come off the posterior ciliary artery, a branch of the ophthalmic artery. SPCAs enter the suprachoroid after only a short oblique course in the sclera and break down into smaller branches to supply extensive choroidal vasculature in a lobular fashion, which is denser in the macular region compared to retinal periphery [52] (Fig. 12). Yoneya and Tso showed the presence of intraarterial and intervenular shunts in the medium-sized vessels in the choroid [38] which may allow some recovery following an ischaemic event or iatrogenic damage during the surgical intervention near the macular area, however, some degree of patchy choroidal ischaemia may be expected.

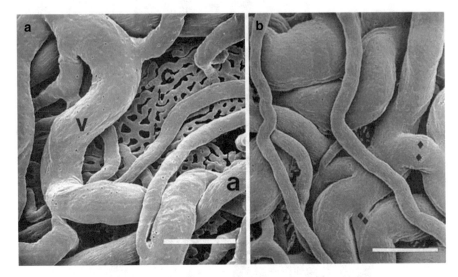

Fig. 12 Scanning electron photograph of a resin cast of the choroidal vasculature showing venules (v), arterioles (a) and choriocapillaris: a- midperiphery (Bar=231μm); b- posterior pole close to fovea (Bar=270 μμlm). (Reproduced with permission from Olver JM, 1990. Eye 1990 ;4 (2):262–7)

Long Posterior Ciliary Arteries (LPCA) Lateral and medial LPCAs are joined by nerves and penetrate the sclera 3–4 mm anterior to the optic nerve and have a longer oblique intrascleral course. They enter the suprachoroidal space posterior to the equator and travel towards the ciliary body and iris root giving off recurrent branches, which loop back to contribute to the macular choriocapillaris, before merging with the major arterial circle at the iris root (Fig. 13).

Vortex Veins The vortex veins have prominent anchoring positions in the SCS (Fig. 14). The superior vortex veins drain blood from the ciliary body and choroid into the superior ophthalmic vein and the corresponding inferior veins into the inferior ophthalmic vein. The vortex pools are usually, but not always, separated by vertical and horizontal landmarks. There are some anatomical variations to the number, diameter, position, and configuration of the vortex veins. The number of vortex veins may vary from 3 to 15, but the most common arrangement is one or two vortex veins in each quadrant exiting the sclera near 1, 5, 7, 11 o'clock positions [46, 53]. The vortex veins are easily identified on fundoscopy just posterior to the equator but may be less obvious in a more pigmented, younger, and more densely vascularised choroid. The inferotemporal quadrant has the highest number of vortex veins. The visible whirling pattern correlates with a larger vortex pool area and a smaller number of vortex systems. A line joining the anterior end of vortex veins indicates the equator of the eyeball. Four patterns of vortex vein formations have been described depending on the point of convergence of tributaries [46] (Fig. 15). This convergence can happen in advance of entering the scleral canal with fully formed ampulla(e); just before entering the scleral canal (no ampulla); whilst entering the sclera (partially formed vortex vein travels together with tributaries) or

Fig. 13 Methyl methacrylate casting of human choroid showing lateral long posterior ciliary artery (black arrow) and recurrent choroidal branch of lateral long posterior ciliary artery (empty arrow) (Reproduced with permission from Olver JM. Functional anatomy of the choroidal circulation. Eye 1990;4 (2):262–72)

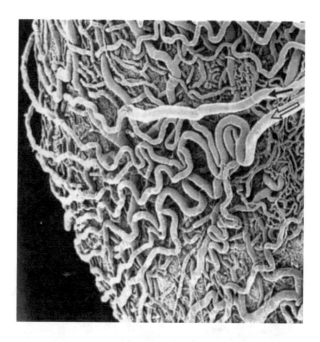

Fig. 14 Scanning electron photomicrograph of a cast of choroidal vasculature showing vortex vein (VV). (Reproduced with permission from Forrester, J. V. et al. The Eye, Basic Sciences in Practice. 4th Edition. Elsevier Ltd. 2015)

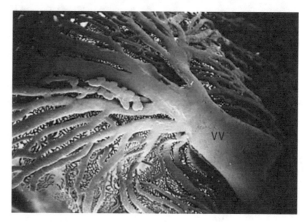

within the sclera and orbit (tributaries enter sclera separately without formed vortex vein). Vortex vein ampullae are seen in a third of examined eyes, having a length of 1–4 mm and an oval shape or that of a tree stump. Exit points of vortex veins are marked by a pigmented crescent and are situated within two disc diameters or 2.5–3.5 mm behind the equator [31].

Ruskell has described choroidopial veins found within approximately 100μm from the optic nerve, an alternative minor route for posterior choroidal drainage directly into the pia mater with a negligible course in the SCS [54].

Lymphatic System The presence of a lymphatic system and uveolymphatic out-flow pathway in the posterior segment of the human eye has been debated [55–58].

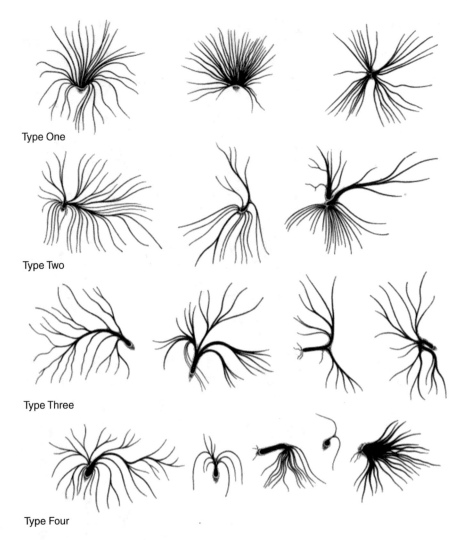

Fig. 15 Four patterns of vortex veins observed by fundoscopy. (Reproduced with permission from Ruthin, 1967 [46])

Histological studies showed evidence of lymphatic vessels in the avian choroid and some mammals [59, 60]. However, human studies found no lymphatic vessels but identified macrophage-like cells with lymphatic endothelial markers in the choroid, e.g. lymphatic vessel endothelial hyaluronic acid receptor (LYVE-1 or podoplanin) and lymphangiogenic factors (VEGF-C) [58, 61–63]. These cannot be referred to as a choroidal lymphatic system based on the consensus for the need of two or more lymphatic markers to be colocalised in the same structures [64].

The role of these cells is not fully understood, and their possible role in pathologic inflammatory conditions awaits further investigation. Development of new ciliary lymphatic channels has been shown in malignancy, suggesting that they may contribute to the lymphogenic spread of ciliary body melanomas and even have prognostic value for the ocular tumour progression and metastasis [65, 66]. Herwig et al. investigated the possibility of a transient intraocular lymphatic system or progenitor vessels during the embryogenesis but found no such evidence in foetal eyes during 10–38 weeks of gestation [67].

Nerves in the Suprachoroid

The suprachoroid hosts a network of fine nerve fibres. Electron microscopic studies showed that ciliary nerves lose their myelin sheath before entering the suprachoroid, where all nerves are therefore unmyelinated [68]. Extensive nerve supply of the choroidal vasculature contributes to autonomous control independent from intraocular and systemic blood pressures. Two groups of nerves that feed this network are the long and short posterior ciliary nerves (synonymous with long and short ciliary nerves respectively). Ciliary ganglion is situated in the superotemporal aspect of the retrobulbar optic nerve approximately 10 mm behind the globe [49, 69]. Also, solitary ganglion cells are scattered in the suprachoroid as well as choroid [27] (Fig. 7). They are collectively referred to as intrinsic choroidal neurons and possibly contribute to smooth muscle cells' control.

Short posterior ciliary nerves (SPCN) emerge from the ciliary ganglion in the number of 10–15 and piercing the sclera around the optic nerve in a ring which is denser superiorly. Their intrascleral course is short and oblique, entering around 2–3 mm from the optic nerve sheath but emerging in the SCS 1–2 mm further, radiating away from the optic nerve [1] (Fig. 16). They travel anteriorly breaking into

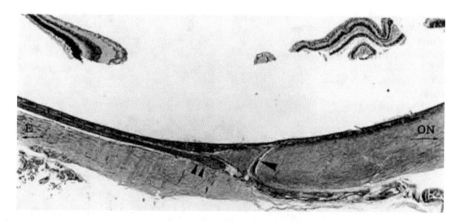

Fig. 16 Emissary canal in sclera for the temporal long posterior ciliary artery and nerve (double arrowhead). Submacular arterial branch (arrowhead) curves posteriorly to enter choroid at a sharp angle and enter SCS obliquely. *E* equator, *ON* optic nerve.(H & E, × 31) (Reproduced with permission from R. Buggage et al, [1])

smaller branches during their course and provide parasympathetic, sympathetic, and sensory supply to the eye.

Sympathetic fibres responsible for vasoconstriction of arterioles travel from superior cervical ganglion through the ciliary ganglion without synapsing and via SPCN provide rich supply to the uveal vessels. A small branch of this nerve innervates Muller's muscle of the upper lid without entering the eyeball. Damage to these fibres usually much earlier in their course causes Horner's syndrome.

Parasympathetic fibres from the Edinger-Westphal nucleus of the oculomotor nerve synapse in the ciliary ganglion before entering the SCS with SPCN to supply the ciliary muscle (accommodation) and the sphincter papillae (miosis). Damage to these fibres (laser or cryo retinopexy) may cause iatrogenic mydriasis and paralysis of accommodation [70]. Parasympathetic fibres responsible for vasodilation, travel with nasociliary nerve from the pterygopalatine ganglion of the facial nerve bypass the ciliary ganglion, enter the SCS either with SPCN or rami oculares that travel along the posterior ciliary arteries [7]. They also innervate nonvascular smooth muscle cells scattered in the suprachoroidal space, but most numerously in the posterior pole and are thought to be synchronous with accommodative action of the ciliary muscle [24].

Sensory innervation Afferent sensory fibres from iris, ciliary body and choroid form the sensory root of the ciliary ganglion, which joins nasociliary nerve [7].

Long posterior ciliary nerves (LPCN)—usually two (nasal and temporal, also referred to as medial and lateral), occasionally three LPCN enter sclera 4–5 mm away from the optic disc in horizontal meridia (~3 and 9 o'clock), traverse sclera obliquely with a longer intrascleral course than SPCN and enter SCS 6–7 mm away from the disc (Fig. 17). Nerve fibres of LPCN bypass ciliary ganglion and do

Fig. 17 Dissected suprachoroidal space of human eye in the macular region with temporal long posterior ciliary nerve. *SPCA* short posterior ciliary arteries, *SPCN* short posterior ciliary nerves, *LPCN* long posterior ciliary nerves

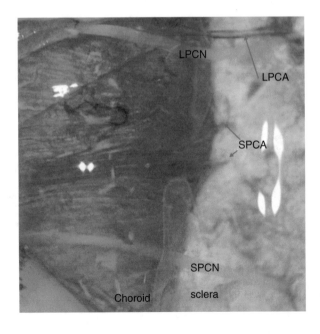

not contain parasympathetic but carry sensory and sympathetic fibres. Some of the fibres from LPCN loop back to supply the anterior choroidal vasculature.

Sympathetic fibres travel from superior cervical ganglion through the ciliary ganglion without synapsing to supply pupil dilator muscle.

Sensory Innervation. Afferent sensory fibres are carried from the anterior segment (cornea, iris and ciliary muscle) to the trigeminal ganglion.

Supraciliary Space

Is continuous with the suprachoroidal space and has similar structural components. Long ciliary nerves travelling in the suprachoroidal space enter the supraciliary space before diving into the ciliary body and iris. The multi-layered collagen lamellae in the supraciliary space become gradually reduced in number and diminished at the scleral spur, it's anterior border [27]. Presence of a compact zone in the supraciliary space has been described in hamster eyes [71], but was not found in primate or human eyes [32, 47].

Topographic Anatomy for Interventive Procedures

The loose attachment of the sclera to the choroid anteriorly allows for relatively effortless entry into the anterior SCS. Any further movement towards the posterior pole is met with some resistance offered by numerous vessels and nerves crossing the SCS (Fig. 18). A small amount of viscoelastic injected into the SCS allows safe advancement, providing the major anatomical landmarks are avoided. When considering the entry point into the SCS, one must be mindful of the horizontal meridia where the long ciliary artery and nerves travel. The scleral curvature can be used to the advantage of the surgeon by letting the cannula or the catheter gently slide along the smooth inner surface of the relatively stiff collagenous sclera. When navigating the instrument in the post-equatorial suprachoroidal space, positions of the vortex ampullae at approximately 11, 1, 5 and 7 o'clock are best avoided. The variation in the number and position of vortex veins can usually be confirmed by fundoscopy before the intervention. The majority of the peripheral breaks in retinal detachment are pre-equatorial and, therefore, easily accessible when approached through sclerotomy 5–6 mm behind the limbus in the clock hour of the break. When considering an intervention in the suprachoroidal space for the breaks overlying the horizontal meridia, one must be aware of the potential effect of distention of SCS on the artery and nerve. The clinical experience suggests that severe pain suffered by patients with acute SCH may be due to stretched ciliary nerve across the SCS. The extent of nerve stretch within the SCS that can be comfortably tolerated by a patient is uncertain and therefore avoiding the ciliary nerves may be advisable.

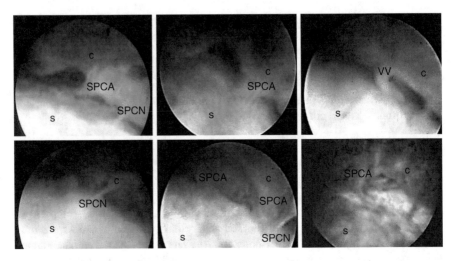

Fig. 18 Endoscopic view of the suprachoroidal space in the macular region. Cloister like spaces are formed between short posterior ciliary arteries and nerves crossing the SCS when distended with viscoelastic. *S* sclera, *C* choroid, *SPCA* short posterior ciliary arteries, *VV* vortex vein, *SPCN* short posterior ciliary nerves

Consideration of the globe's configuration is important when planning intervention in the SCS of the eye with pathologic myopia especially at the outpouching edge of staphyloma, where the radius of curvature changes, to prevent damage to retina and choroid.

Suprachoroidal Space and Uveal Effusion

Patients with hypermetropia and nanophthalmos (axial length <21 mm) may have impaired transscleral outflow and develop uveal effusion syndrome (UES), a condition associated with accumulation of fluid in the SCS [72]. The disorganisation of collagen fibres and deposition of proteoglycan debris between them are seen on histologic samples of sclerae from affected eyes [73]. Possible mechanisms for choroidal effusions are compression of vortex veins and transscleral emissaria by the thickened sclera and impaired scleral permeability. The hypothesis that UES is caused by impaired hydraulic conductivity of abnormal sclera has been rejected by Jackson et al. [73]. They investigated the scleral permeability ex vivo and proposed that the fluid is retained in the suprachoroidal space by colloid osmotic forces. They found increased rather than decreased the hydraulic conductivity of the sclerae from the eyes with uveal effusion, but reduced the transport of macromolecules, leading to retained protein and increased oncotic pressure within the SCS due to an accumulation of albumin [39, 73, 74].

Forrester et al. suggested that the UES is due to a primary defect in proteodermatan synthesis and/or degradation by scleral fibroblasts and may represent a form of ocular mucopolysaccharidosis [75].

Suprachoroid in High Myopia

Myopia is referred to as pathologic when the axial length exceeds 26.5 mm, and the refraction is worse than −8.0 D [14]. In most high myopes the eye develops normally through the gestation, but progressive scleral thinning and ocular expansion occur during the childhood, leading to further abnormalities of the underlying choroid and retina [14] and therefore inevitably in the suprachoroid. The sclera may undergo extensive changes, such as thinning, change in the curvature with localised outpouchings (staphylomas), widening of the emissary openings, and tilting and distortion of the scleral canal [14].

In the choroid, thinning and patchy disappearance is observed with a loss of the overlying RPE and outer retina. The atrophic patches enlarge with time, resulting in broad white areas of the absent choroid. These correlate with pathologic findings in the sclera [15]. In the areas of chorioretinal atrophy, the SCS merges with the subretinal space.

The oblique course of emissary vessels in the thinned distorted sclera can become shorter and enlargement of the internal openings of the emissary channels can be observed [14]. These can be visible on fundoscopy and OCT as a funnel-shaped depression or intrascleral cavitation associated with attenuated vessels and possibly with a full-thickness defect in eyes with extensive atrophy of the choroid, RPE and overlying retina [76]. They can be found near the optic nerve or away from the nerve [14] (Fig. 19).

Suprachoroidal Changes with Age

Several molecular changes take place in the sclera with age. The cross-linking between collagen fibres and glycosylation with an accumulation of end products increases [77]. The sclera becomes stiffer due to reduction of collagen and elastin fibres, decline in their diameter and regularity, and content of glycosaminoglycans, leading to reduced hydration [78–83]. The choroid also undergoes extensive changes which include thinning, and also cracking of the thickened Bruch's membrane. Consequently, with thinning of choroidal tissue and impaired hydration of the sclera, SCS widens with age, evident on the EDI OCT and histological sections [42].

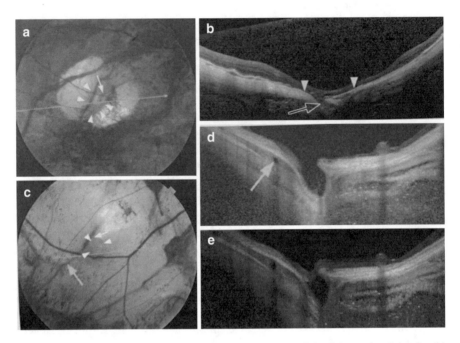

Fig. 19 Scleral emissary openings in a highly myopic eye (**a**) Scleral depression (arrowheads) with a blood vessel (arrow); (**b**) corresponding OCT scan shows the enlarged emissary passageway (open arrow) with a full-thickness defect in thinned sclera; (**c**) A circular scleral depression (arrowheads) has absent choroid and visible deeper vessel (arrow); (**d**) OCT shows cross section of the depression along the green line with arrow pointing at the vessel in (**c**); (**e**) OCT was taken slightly inferior to the above OCT and shows retina draping across the scleral opening. (Reproduced with permission from Spaide, R [14])

Physiology

The suprachoroid plays an important role in maintaining normal fluid dynamics within an eye. The ECM of the suprachoroid between collagen and elastic fibres is filled with plasma-like fluid and glycosaminoglycans, including hyaluronic acid [1, 27].

Fluid accumulated in the suprachoroidal space can arrive there from several sources:

- Anterior chamber - aqueous humour travels between the fibres of the ciliary muscle and the supraciliary space (unconventional aqueous outflow)
- Choroidal vasculature
- Periocular space transsclerally

These can be triggered by and exaggerated in pathological conditions such as iris dialysis, exudation from impaired choroidal vasculature, ocular hypotony or scleral abnormality.

The outflow of the fluid from the SCS occurs in two directions:

- Uveoscleral outflow (trans-scleral migration and bulk flow around the emissaria)
- Uveovortex outflow (fluid is absorbed by choriocapillaris into the vortex veins)

A uveo-lymphatic pathway was proposed after discovering dual lymphatic endothelial vascular markers in the ciliary body which may contribute to aqueous drainage [58]. These findings were not reproduced in a similar study, and therefore such outflow is unlikely to be present in physiological conditions [84].

Uveoscleral Outflow

The main pathway for the drainage of aqueous from the anterior chamber is the conventional or trabecular outflow through the trabecular meshwork into the episcleral veins via Schlemm's canal and the collector channels.

The other aqueous drainage pathway discovered later and therefore named "unconventional," is from the anterior chamber into the supraciliary and suprachoroidal space, through the ciliary muscle between its longitudinal fibres [85]. Although the term uveoscleral has become synonymous with unconventional outflow, a more accurate term perhaps would have been suprachoroidal outflow as it embraces not only uveoscleral but also uveovortex paths.

Anders Bill was the first to develop the methods to study unconventional outflow's route and rate. In his extensive investigations [41, 85–95] he has described the uveoscleral outflow to be independent from intraocular pressure (IOP) in primates [87] and constituted 4–14% of the total aquous outflow in human eye [41]. When treated with atropine, the flow increased up to 27% [41]; and in eyes treated with pilocarpine, it was reduced to 0–3% [87]. Furthermore, 1.2% of radiolabelled albumin was found in the vortex vein [41] via uveovortex outflow [96, 97]. A more recent detailed summary of variations in measurements of unconventional uveal outflow was made by Johnson et al., and outflow varied from 0–1.52µl/min which constituted 0–85% of aqueous inflow and was found to be higher in younger adults compared to older adults [98, 99]. This finding was backed by morphologic studies showing the build-up of connective tissue between ciliary muscle fibres with age [100].

The uveal outflow occurs passively as there is no epithelial barrier between the anterior chamber and the ciliary muscle. However, the presence of several layers of intertwined cells with junctional complexes between the fibroblasts of the suprachoroid [32] may offer some, however small, resistance to the drainage.

The ciliary muscle appears to be the main point of resistance. Cholinergic contraction of the ciliary muscle reduces the outflow into the suprachoroid. In contrast, relaxation of the ciliary muscle increases the drainage into SCS due to widening of spaces between muscle bundles [41, 94]. Epinephrine, β-adrenergic drug, increases uveoscleral outflow in monkeys; although the exact mechanism was not known [90]. Matrix metalloproteinases (MMP) are found to contribute to the uveoscleral outflow regulation [51]. Prostaglandins are shown to increase uveal outflow by promoting secretion of MMP and remodelling the extracellular matrix causing loss of collagen fibres between the ciliary muscle fibres [101, 102].

Although constant and insensitive to the fluctuation of IOP, the outflow via uveal outflow pathway increases when the trabecular resistance increases, but the exact adaptive mechanisms for this are not yet understood.

Fluid Dynamics in the Eye and the Suprachoroidal Space

A fine balance of intraocular fluid inflow and outflow is maintained by a complex collaboration of obvious and more subtle mechanisms. The uvea is the main source of fluid, i.e. ciliary body secretion and the leaky choroidal vasculature. The less obvious one is the eyeball's external wall- the corneal endothelium pump and non-discriminate bidirectional hydraulic conductivity of the sclera. The latter is in an outward direction in physiological conditions due to pressure gradient but may reverse with the ocular hypotony. The outflow routes are mainly via trabecular meshwork and unconventional route via suprachoroid. The latter is governed by the hydrostatic pressure in the SCS.

Emi et al. attempted to measure the hydrostatic pressure of the eye at three points of primate eyes: the anterior chamber, the supraciliary space and the SCS at the equator [40]. They found that the hydrostatic pressure in the posterior SCS was 3.5–4.2 mm lower than that in the anterior chamber (i.e. IOP) and 2.6–3.3 mm lower than that in the supraciliary space. This pressure gradient is believed to determine the direction of flow. An increase in IOP from 15 to 60 mmHg led to a proportional elevation of hydrostatic pressure in both the supraciliary space and the SCS. The elevation was consistently around 1 mm below IOP in the supraciliary space, but was less consistent and up to 10 mm lower than IOP in the SCS. This trend was also true for the lower-than-normal IOP. Lowering the pressure to 4 mm for longer than 20 min caused a drop to negative pressure in the SCS. These findings showed that the pressure in the SCS is not insensitive to IOP; instead, it increases and decreases with it but at a slower rate. The anatomical explanation for such a difference in the pressure has not been fully elucidated. Presence of compact zone in the supraciliary space was described in hamster eyes but was not found in primate eyes [47, 71]. One possible explanation for the pressure difference is the presence of several layers of tightly packed fibroblasts and melanocytes with junctional complexes, offering some resistance to the drainage both into and out of the SCS.

An in-vivo study measured outflow via SCS to be 1.1–1.5μL/min [99]. An ex-vivo study estimated scleral outflow to be three times higher at 4.3μL/min [74]. This potential for higher drainage is realised in the clinical scenario of cyclodialysis and secondary ocular hypotony. It supports the suggestion that ciliary muscle is the main gateway into the SCS.

An interesting observation was the development of negative pressure in the SCS with the sudden drop of IOP from 60 to 4 mmHg [40]. Orbital (extraocular) pressure was estimated to be around 3–6 mmHg in normal conditions [103]; therefore, for negative pressure to be created, an active pump is required. This cannot be achieved with scleral conductivity alone, and choroidal capillaries are the most likely to act as an active pump. In cases of persistent hypotony, for example, after trabeculectomy, a reversal in the direction of the flow and accumulation of transudate in the SCS, i.e. choroidal effusion may occur (see Chapter "Choroidal Detachment"). In the context of an open globe injury, this may lead to overstretch and rupture of the vessels crossing the SCS, leading to suprachoroidal haemorrhage (see Chapter "Suprachoroidal Choroidal Haemorrhage").

The inward absorption of drugs administered into the peribulbar space of a normotensive eye may be counteracted by transscleral aqueous outflow. The scleral conductivity for small molecules was not influenced by the thickness of the sclera, but was reduced for larger molecules [39, 73].

The oncotic pressure, or colloid osmotic pressure, is generated by plasma proteins, mainly albumin. The extravascular uveal albumin concentration depends on the capillary permeability and its reabsorption by choriocapillaris and transscleral conductivity. The capillaries of the ciliary body and choroid are fenestrated, allowing extravasation of protein. The choriocapillaris appears to be more discriminate in the size of protein they will allow out [104, 105], possibly explaining the difference in the hydrostatic pressure between supraciliary and suprachoroidal spaces.

Emi et al. found over a three-fold difference in the protein concentration between the SCS (23.7 mg/ml) and the plasma (82.1 mg/ml) when measured in vivo in primates [40]. In the extravascular choroid of a monkey, the effective albumin concentration was <13% of plasma [105]. They suggested that this colloid osmotic pressure difference is the main driver for the fluid absorption from the SCS by gradient across the choriocapillaris. A collection of suprachoroidal fluid in physiological conditions is technically difficult, but was measured in pathological condition. The transudate in choroidal effusions contained protein molecules no larger than 150 K Da, suggesting the sieving limit of choriocapillaris pores [104].

The colloid osmotic pressure difference is nearly constant in normal circumstances, and the hydrostatic pressure governs the direction of serum protein. Consequently, the high hydrostatic pressure in the SCS prevents the serum protein leakage and keeps the protein concentration lower, facilitating the fluid outflow from the SCS [40]. In pathological conditions with low hydrostatic pressure in the SCS, the opposite must take place. Serum protein leak occurs, increasing the protein concentration in the SCS and decreasing the outflow of the suprachoroidal fluid. The result is a smaller pressure difference between the SCS and the anterior chamber. This can be seen as a compensatory mechanism for reducing the uveoscleral outflow in a hypotonous eye.

Summary

In this chapter, we have reviewed the anatomy and physiology of the suprachoroid in normal eyes and in some pathological conditions as the basis for the interventive procedures discussed in the subsequent chapters. Our investigation tools and the spectrum of interventions are rapidly developing as will our understanding of this fascinating part of the eye.

References

1. Buggage RR, Torzynski E, Grossniklaus H. In: Duane TD, editor. Duane's clinical ophthalmology. Chapter 22 choroid and suprachoroid. Philadelphia, PA: Lipincott, Williams & Wilkins; 2006.
2. Mann I. Development of the human eye. New York: Grune & Stratton; 1964.
3. Sellheyer K, Spitznas M. Development of the human sclera. Graefe's Arch Clin Exp Ophthalmol [Internet]. 1988;226(1):89–100. https://doi.org/10.1007/BF02172725.
4. Anand-Apte B, Hollyfield JG. Developmental anatomy of the retinal and choroidal vasculature. Encycl Eye. 2010:9–15.
5. Fledelius HC, Christensen AC. Reappraisal of the human ocular growth curve in fetal life, infancy, and early childhood. Br J Ophthalmol. 1996;80(10):918–21.
6. Sellheyer K. Development of the choroid and related structures. Eye. 1990;4(2):255–61.
7. Oyster CW. The human eye: structure and function. 1999.
8. Mund ML, Rodrigues MM, Fine BS. Light and electron microscopic observations on the pigmented layers of the developing human eye. Am J Ophthalmol. 1972;73(2):167–82.
9. Olsen TW, Aaberg SY, Geroski DH, Edelhauser HF. Human sclera: thickness and surface area. Am J Ophthalmol. 1998;125(2):237–41.
10. Spitznas M. The fine structure of human scleral collagen. Am J Ophthalmol. 1971;71(1):68.
11. Watson P, Hazleman B, McCluskey P, Pavésio C. Anatomical, physiological, and comparative aspects. In: The sclera and systemic disorders. Jaypee Brothers Medical Publishers (P) Ltd.; 2012. p. 11–45. https://www.jaypeedigital.com/book/9781907816079/chapter/ch2.
12. Rada JA, Achen VR, Perry CA, Fox PW. Proteoglycans in the human sclera. Evidence for the presence of aggrecan. Invest Ophthalmol Vis Sci. 1997;38(9):1740–51.
13. Trier K, Olsen EB, Ammitzbøll T. Regional glycosaminoglycans composition of the human sclera. Acta Ophthalmol. 2009;68(3):304–6. https://doi.org/10.1111/j.1755-3768.1990.tb01926.x.
14. Spaide RF, Ohno-Matsui K, Yanuzzi L. Pathologic myopia. 2014.
15. Ohno-Matsui K, Akiba M, Modegi T, Tomita M, Ishibashi T, Tokoro T, et al. Association between shape of sclera and myopic retinochoroidal lesions in patients with pathologic myopia. Investig Ophthalmol Vis Sci. 2012;53(10):6046–61.
16. Parver LM, Auker C, Carpenter DO. Choroidal blood flow as a heat dissipating mechanism in the macula. Am J Ophthalmol. 1980;89(5):641–6.
17. Saint-Geniez M, Maldonado AE, D'Amore PA. VEGF expression and receptor activation in the choroid during development and in the adult. Investig Opthalmology Vis Sci. 2006;47(7):3135. https://doi.org/10.1167/iovs.05-1229.
18. Frank RN, Amin RH, Eliott D, Puklin JE, Abrams GW. Basic fibroblast growth factor and vascular endothelial growth factor are present in epiretinal and choroidal neovascular membranes. Am J Ophthalmol. 1996;122(3):393–403.
19. Grierson I, Heathcote L, Hiscott P, Hogg P, Briggs M, Hagan S. Hepatocyte growth factor/ scatter factor in the eye. Prog Retin Eye Res. 2000;19(6):779–802.
20. Hu W, Criswell MH, Fong S-L, Temm CJ, Rajashekhar G, Cornell TL, et al. Differences in the temporal expression of regulatory growth factors during choroidal neovascular development. Exp Eye Res. 2009;88(1):79–91.
21. Steen B, Sejersen S, Berglin L, Seregard S, Kvanta A. Matrix metalloproteinases and metalloproteinase inhibitors in choroidal neovascular membranes. Invest Ophthalmol Vis Sci. 1998;39(11):2194–200.
22. Ogata N, Matsushima M, Takada Y, Tobe T, Takahashi K, Yi X, et al. Expression of basic fibroblast growth factor mRNA in developing choroidal neovascularization. Curr Eye Res. 1996;15(10):1008–18. https://doi.org/10.3109/02713689609017649.
23. Hayreh SS. In vivo choroidal circulation and its watershed zones. Eye. 1990;4(2):273–89.
24. May CA. Non-vascular smooth muscle cells in the human choroid: distribution, development and further characterization. J Anat. 2005;207(4):381–90. https://doi.org/10.1111/j.1469-7580.2005.00460.x.

25. Poukens V, Glasgow BJ, BJ JLD. Nonvascular contractile cells in sclera and choroid of humans and monkeys. Invest Ophthalmol Vis Sci. 1998;39(10):1765–4.
26. de Hoz R, Ramírez AI, Salazar JJ, Rojas B, Ramírez JM, Triviño A. Substance P and calcitonin gene-related peptide intrinsic choroidal neurons in human choroidal whole-mounts. Histol Histopathol. 2008;23(10):1249–58.
27. Hogan MJ, Alvarado JA, Esperson WJ. Histology of the human eye : an atlas and textbook. Philadelphia, PA: Saunders; 1971.
28. Wolff's anatomy of the eye and orbit. 1991. 371–385 p.
29. Lewis WH. Gray's anatomy of the Human body. Philadelphia and New York: Lea Brothers & Co.; 1918.
30. Gray H, Carter HV. Anatomy descriptive and surgical [Internet]. 1858, pp. 553–554. https://ia802705.us.archive.org/2/items/anatomydescript09graygoog/anatomy-descript09graygoog.pdf
31. Salzmann M. Anatomy and histology of the human eyeball in normal state: its development and senescence. Chicago, IL: Chicago Univercity Press; 1912.
32. Koseki T. Ultrastructural studies of the lamina suprachoroidea in the human eye. Nihon Ganka Gakkai Zasshi. 1992;96(6):757–66.
33. Feeney ABL, Hogan MJ. Electron microscopy of the human choroid. Am J Ophthalmol. 1961;51(5):1057/185–72/200.
34. Olver JM, Mc Cartney ACE. Orbital and ocular micro-vascular corrosion casting in man. Eye. 1989;3(5):588–96.
35. Woodlief NF, Eifrig DE. Initial observations on the ocular microcirculation in man: the choriocapillaris. Ann Ophthalmol. 1982;14(2):176–80.
36. Krohn J, Bertelsen T. Corrosion casts of the suprachoroidal space and uveoscleral drainage routes in the human eye. Acta Ophthalmol Scand. 1997;75(1):32–5. https://doi.org/10.1111/j.1600-0420.1997.tb00245.x.
37. Flower RW, Fryczkowski AW, McLeod DS. Variability in choriocapillaris blood flow distribution. Investig Ophthalmol Vis Sci. 1995;36:1247–58.
38. Yoneya S, Tso MOM. Angioarchitecture of the Human choroid. Arch Ophthalmol. 1987;105(5):681–7.
39. Anderson OA, Jackson TL, Singh JK, Hussain AA, Marshall J. Human transscleral albumin permeability and the effect of topographical location and donor age. Investig Ophthalmol Vis Sci. 2008;49(9):4041–5.
40. Emi K, Pederson JE, Toris CB, Hydrostatic pressure of the suprachoroidal space. Investig Ophthalmol Vis Sci. 1989;30(2):233–8.
41. Bill A, Phillips CI. Uveoscleral drainage of aqueous humour in human eyes. Exp Eye Res. 1971;12(3):275–81.
42. Yiu G, Pecen P, Sarin N, Chiu SJ, Farsiu S, Mruthyunjaya P, et al. Characterization of the choroid-scleral junction and suprachoroidal layer in healthy individuals on enhanced-depth imaging optical coherence tomography. JAMA Ophthalmol. 2014;132(2):174–81.
43. Margolis R, Spaide RF. A pilot study of enhanced depth imaging optical coherence tomography of the choroid in normal eyes. Am J Ophthalmol. 2009;147(5):811–5.
44. Spaide RF, Koizumi H, Pozonni MC. Enhanced depth imaging spectral-domain optical coherence tomography. Am J Ophthalmol. 2008;146(4):496–500.
45. Krohn J, Bertelsen T. Corrosion casts of the suprachoroidal space and uveoscleral drainage routes in the pig eye. Acta Ophthalmol Scand. 1997;75(1):28–31.
46. Rutnin U. Fundus appearance in normal eyes. I choroid. Am J Ophthalmol. 1967;64(5):821–39.
47. Wood RL, Koseki T, Kelly DE. Structural analysis of potential barriers to bulk-flow exchanges between uvea and sclera in eyes of Macaque monkeys. Cell Tissue Res. 1990;260(3):459–68. https://doi.org/10.1007/BF00297225.
48. Nag TC, Kumari C. Electron microscopy of the human choroid. Choroidal Disorders. Elsevier Inc.; 2017. p. 7–20. https://doi.org/10.1016/B978-0-12-805313-3.00002-8.
49. Wolff E. The anatomy of the eye and orbit. London: H.K.Lewis & Co. Ltd.; 1940. p. 41–2.
50. Flügel-Koch C, May CA, Lütjen-Drecoll E. Presence of a contractile cell network in the human choroid. Ophthalmologica. 1996;210(5):296–302.

51. Gaton DD, Sagara T, Lindsey JD, Weinreb RN. Matrix metalloproteinase-1 localization in the normal human uveoscleral outflow pathway. Investig Ophthalmol Vis Sci. 1999;40(2):363–9.
52. Krey HF. Segmental vascular patterns of the choriocapillaris. Am J Ophthalmol. 1975 Aug;80(2):198–202.
53. Ruthin U, Schepens CL. Fundus appearance in normal eyes. II The standard peripheral fundus and developmental variations. Am J Ophthalmol. 1967;64(5):840–52.
54. Ruskell GL. Peripapillary venous drainage from the choroid: a variable feature in human eyes. Br J Ophthalmol. 1997;81(1):77–9.
55. Lutty GA. Adult human choroid: an alymphatic tissue? Investig Opthalmology Vis Sci. 2015;56(12):7417. https://doi.org/10.1167/iovs.15-18531.
56. Grüntzig J, Hollmann F. Lymphatic vessels of the eye - old questions - new insights. Ann Anat. 2019;221:1–16.
57. Nakao S, Hafezi-Moghadam A, Ishibashi T. Lymphatics and lymphangiogenesis in the eye. J Ophthalmol. 2012;2012:1–11.
58. Yücel YH, Johnston MG, Ly T, Patel M, Drake B, Gümüş E, et al. Identification of lymphatics in the ciliary body of the human eye: a novel "uveolymphatic" outflow pathway. Exp Eye Res. 2009;89(5):810–9.
59. De Stefano ME, Mugnaini E. Fine structure of the choroidal coat of the avian eye. Vascularization, supporting tissue and innervation. Anat Embryol (Berl). 1997;195(5):393–418.
60. Krebs W. Ultrastructural evidence for lymphatic capillaries in the primate choroid. Arch Ophthalmol. 1988;106(11):1615. https://doi.org/10.1001/archopht.1988.01060140783055.
61. Schrödl F, Kaser-Eichberger A, Trost A, Strohmaier C, Bogner B, Runge C, et al. Lymphatic markers in the adult human choroid. Investig Opthalmology Vis Sci. 2015;56(12):7406. https://doi.org/10.1167/iovs.15-17883.
62. Koina ME, Baxter L, Adamson SJ, Arfuso F, Hu P, Madigan MC, et al. Evidence for lymphatics in the developing and adult human choroid. Invest Ophthalmol Vis Sci. 2015;56(2):1310–27. https://doi.org/10.1167/iovs.14-15705.
63. Schroedl F, Brehmer A, Neuhuber WL, Kruse FE, May CA, Cursiefen C. The normal human choroid is endowed with a significant number of lymphatic vessel endothelial hyaluronate receptor 1 (LYVE-1)–positive macrophages. Investig Opthalmology Vis Sci. 2008;49(12):5222. https://doi.org/10.1167/iovs.08-1721.
64. Schroedl F, Kaser-Eichberger A, Schlereth SL, Bock F, Regenfuss B, Reitsamer HA, et al. Consensus statement on the immunohistochemical detection of ocular lymphatic vessels. Invest Ophthalmol Vis Sci. 2014;55(10):6440–2.
65. Heindl LM. Intraocular lymphatics in ciliary body melanomas with extraocular extension. Arch Ophthalmol. 2010;128(8):1001. https://doi.org/10.1001/archophthalmol.2010.143.
66. Heindl LM, Hofmann TN, Adler W, Knorr HLJ, Holbach LM, Naumann GOH, et al. Intraocular tumor-associated Lymphangiogenesis. Ophthalmology. 2010;117(2):334–42.
67. Herwig MC, Münstermann K, Klarmann-Schulz U, Schlereth SL, Heindl LM, Loeffler KU, et al. Expression of the lymphatic marker podoplanin (D2-40) in human fetal eyes. Exp Eye Res. 2014;127:243–51.
68. Feeney L, Hogan MJ. Electron microscopy of the human choroid. II. The choroidal nerves. Am J Ophthalmol. 1961;51(5):1084–212.
69. Dutton JJ. Orbital nerves. Atlas Clin Surg Orbital Anat. 2011:51–82.
70. Kaufman PL, Rohen JW, Gabelt BT, Eichhorn M, Wallow IHL, Polansky JR. Parasympathetic denervation of the ciliary muscle following panretinal photocoagulation. Curr Eye Res. 1991;10(5):437–55.
71. Kelly DE, Hageman GS, McGregor JA. Uveal compartmentalization in the hamster eye revealed by fine structural and tracer studies: implications for uveoscleral outflow. Invest Ophthalmol Vis Sci. 1983;24(9):1288–304.
72. Uyama M, Takahashi K, Kozaki J, Tagami N, Takada Y, Ohkuma H, et al. Uveal effusion syndrome: clinical features, surgical treatment, histologic examination of the sclera, and pathophysiology. Ophthalmology. 2000;107(3):441–9.

73. Jackson TL, Hussain A, AMS M, Sullivan PM, Hodgetts A, El-Osta A, et al. Scleral hydraulic conductivity and macromolecular diffusion in patients with uveal effusion syndrome. Investig Ophthalmol Vis Sci. 2008;49(11):5033–40.
74. Jackson TL, Hussain A, Hodgetts A, Morley AMS, Hillenkamp J, Sullivan PM, et al. Human scleral hydraulic conductivity: age-related changes, topographical variation, and potential scleral outflow facility. Invest Ophthalmol Vis Sci. 2006;47(11):4942–6.
75. Forrester JV, Lee WR, Kerr PR, Dua HS. The uveal effusion syndrome and trans-scleral flow. Eye (Lond). 1990;4(Pt 2):354–65.
76. Ohno-Matsui K, Akiba M, Moriyama M, Ishibashi T, Hirakata A, Tokoro T. Intrachoroidal cavitation in macular area of eyes with pathologic myopia. Am J Ophthalmol. 2012;154(2):382–93.
77. Renwick Beattie J, Pawlak AM, McGarvey JJ, Stitt AW. Sclera as a surrogate marker for determining AGE-modifications in Bruch's membrane using a raman spectroscopy-based index of aging. Investig Ophthalmol Vis Sci. 2011;52(3):1593–8.
78. Watson PG, Young RD. Scleral structure, organisation and disease. A review. Exp Eye Res. 2004;78(3):609–23.
79. Rada JA, Achen VR, Penugonda S, Schmidt RW, Mount BA. Proteoglycan composition in the human sclera during growth and aging. Investig Ophthalmol Vis Sci. 2000;41(7):1639–48.
80. Brown CT, Vural M, Johnson M, Trinkaus-Randall V. Age-related changes of scleral hydration and sulfated glycosaminoglycans. Mech Ageing Dev. 1994;77(2):97–107.
81. Geraghty B, Jones SW, Rama P, Akhtar R, Elsheikh A. Age-related variations in the biomechanical properties of human sclera. J Mech Behav Biomed Mater. 2012;16:181–91.
82. Girard MJA, Suh JKF, Bottlang M, Burgoyne CF, Downs JC. Scleral biomechanics in the aging monkey eye. Investig Ophthalmol Vis Sci. 2009;50(11):5226–37.
83. Elsheikh A, Geraghty B, Alhasso D, Knappett J, Campanelli M, Rama P. Regional variation in the biomechanical properties of the human sclera. Exp Eye Res. 2010;90(5):624–33.
84. Kaser-Eichberger A, Schrödl F, Trost A, Strohmaier C, Bogner B, Runge C, et al. Topography of lymphatic markers in human iris and ciliary body. Investig Opthalmology Vis Sci. 2015;56(8):4943. https://doi.org/10.1167/iovs.15-16573.
85. Bill A, Hellsing K. Production and drainage of aqueous humor in the cynomolgus monkey (Macaca irus). Invest Ophthalmol. 1965;4(5):920–6.
86. Bill A. Further studies on the influence of the intraocular pressure on aqueous humor dynamics in cynomolgus monkeys. Investig Ophthalmol Vis Sci. 1967;6(4):364–72.
87. Bill A, Walinder P-E. The effects of pilocarpine on the dynamics of aqueous humor in a primate (Macaca irus). Invest Ophthalmol Vis Scinvestigative Ophthalmol Vis Sci. 1966;5:170–5.
88. Alm A, Bill A. Ocular and optic nerve blood flow at normal and increased intraocular pressures in monkeys (Macaca irus): a study with radioactively labelled microspheres including flow determinations in brain and some other tissues. Exp Eye Res. 1973;15(1):15–29.
89. Bill A. Aqueous humor dynamics in monkeys (Macaca irus and Cercopithecus ethiops). Exp Eye Res. 1971;11(2):195–206.
90. Bill A. Effects of norepinephrine, isoproterenol and sympathetic stimulation on aqueous humour dynamics in vervet monkeys. Exp Eye Res. 1970;10(1):31–46.
91. Bill A. Uveoscleral drainage of aqueous humor: physiology and pharmacology. Prog Clin Biol Res. 1989;312:417–27.
92. Bill A. Some aspects of aqueous humour drainage. Eye. 1993;7(1):14–9.
93. Bill A. Blood circulation and fluid dynamics in the eye. Physiol Rev. 1975;55(3):383–417. https://doi.org/10.1152/physrev.1975.55.3.383.
94. Nilsson SF. The uveoscleral outflow routes. Eye. 1997;11(2):149–54.
95. Bill A. The drainage of albumin from the uvea. Exp Eye Res. 1964;3:179–87.
96. Pederson JE, Gaasterland DE, MacLellan HM. Uveoscleral aqueous outflow in the rhesus monkey: importance of uveal reabsorption. Investig Ophthalmol Vis Sci. 1977;16(11):1008–17.
97. Sherman SH, Green K, Laties AM. The fate of anterior chamber fluorescein in the monkey eye 1. The anterior chamber outflow pathways. Exp Eye Res. 1978;27(2):159–73.

98. Johnson M, McLaren JW, Overby DR. Unconventional aqueous humor outflow: A review. Exp Eye Res. 2017;158:94–111.
99. Toris CB, Yablonski ME, Wang YL, Camras CB. Aqueous humor dynamics in the aging human eye. Am J Ophthalmol. 1999;127(4):407–12.
100. Tamm S, Tamm E, Rohen JW. Age-related changes of the human ciliary muscle. A quantitative morphometric study. Mech Ageing Dev. 1992;62(2):209–21.
101. Lindsey JD, Kashiwagi K, Boyle D, Kashiwagi F, Firestein GS, Weinreb RN. Prostaglandins increase proMMP-1 and proMMP-3 secretion by human ciliary smooth muscle cells. Curr Eye Res. 1996;15(8):869–75. https://doi.org/10.3109/02713689609017628.
102. Lütjen-Drecoll E, Tamm E. Morphological study of the anterior segment of cynomolgus monkey eyes following treatment with prostaglandin F2α. Exp Eye Res. 1988;47(5):761–9.
103. Kratky V, Hurwitz JJ, Avram DR. Orbital compartment syndrome. Direct measurement of orbital tissue pressure: 1. Technique. Can J Ophthalmol. 1990;25(6):293–7.
104. Chylack LT, Bellows AR. Molecular sieving in suprachoroidal fluid formation in man. Invest Ophthalmol Vis Sci. 1978;17(5):420–7.
105. Toris CB, Pederson JE, Tsuboi S, Gregerson DS, Rice TJ. Extravascular albumin concentration of the uvea. Invest Ophthalmol Vis Sci. 1990;31(1):43–53.

Imaging the Suprachoroidal Space

Richard F. Spaide and Yale Fisher

Introduction

The choroid has a high density of blood vessels embedded in an extracellular matrix which is composed of collagen and ground substance. With increasing age, the amount of ground substance appears to decrease, resulting in changes in the packing of the collagen [1, 2]. This has been theorised to produce changes in the structural, optical coherence tomography (OCT) appearance of the choroid. There is a polarisation of vessel sizes in the choroid, with the choriocapillaris along the inner surface and the large Haller's vessels dominating the outer portion of the choroid. In between are the medium sized vessels termed Sattler's layer. The medium and large vessels may be intermixed, so there is often no "layer" appearance. In addition to intervening collagen and ground substance, there are interspersed melanocytes.

The sclera is the tough fibrous, protective shell of the eye. The bulk of the sclera is formed by interwoven fibres of predominantly Type 1 collagen. These fibres are embedded in an extracellular matrix containing glycosaminoglycans, the type of which varies regionally in the sclera [3].

On the inner surface of the sclera is the suprachoroidea, which is approximately 30 μm thick [4]. The suprachoroidea contains collagen fibres, melanocytes, fibroblasts, ganglion cells and nerve plexuses [4]. The exact plane of splitting in the formation of the suprachoroidal space is not known with certainty. In some eyes, it may be in the suprachoroidea and in others in front of the suprachoroidea. This potential space may be expanded by exudation, blood, medications [5–7], and mechanical devices [8]. Imaging the suprachoroidal space provides an opportunity to diagnose abnormalities, monitor the progress of healing, evaluate drug dosing and distribution, appraise the positioning of implanted cannulas and devices, and potentially locate foreign bodies.

R. F. Spaide (✉) · Y. Fisher
Vitreous, Retina, Macula Consultants of New York, New York, NY, USA

© The Author(s), under exclusive license to Springer Nature Switzerland AG 2021
S. Saidkasimova, T. H. Williamson (eds.), *Suprachoroidal Space Interventions*,
https://doi.org/10.1007/978-3-030-76853-9_2

Methods of Imaging the Suprachoroidal Space

The principal methods of imaging the suprachoroidal space in clinical practice employ either contact B-scan ultrasonography or optical coherence tomography. There are other methods that have utility, even if they are not practised as commonly. Simple observation of transillumination can help differentiate an anterior staphyloma from a choroidal tumour invading and distorting the sclera. Magnetic resonance imaging and computed tomography can be used to evaluate the suprachoroidal space for foreign bodies and drug distribution [9–11]. Radiologic imaging may have a theoretical advantage in severely disrupted globes because there is no need for either contact or clear media to gain useful imaging. Otherwise, contact B-scan ultrasonography and OCT have greater clinical utility, expediency, and lower cost.

Contact B-Scan Ultrasonography

An ultrasonic probe typically uses a piezoelectric crystal as a transducer, which is a component that converts one form of energy to another. Initially, the piezoelectric crystal is stimulated electronically to generate an ultrasonic pulse, which radiates into a tissue. The electric field then is removed from the piezo crystal. Any returning reflections from the tissue can cause the crystal to vibrate, which causes the transducer to generate an electric field in proportion to the deformation of the piezo element.

Ultrasonic pulses travel through tissue and can be reflected by tissue planes. The magnitude of the reflection is related to the angle of incidence and the relationship between the acoustic impedance of the media on either side of the interface. Snell's law can be used to calculate how obliquely incident wavefronts are refracted at the interface in the media. Sound energy also meets resistance to its passage through tissue. Some of this resistance is due to the elasticity of the media and is called acoustic reactance. The other part is due to loss of sound energy as it is converted to heat and is called acoustic resistance. The proportion of sound energy lost is complicated to calculate but is related to the different molecular relaxation processes that may occur in various materials and a power law relationship with the frequency of the sound.

The simple carry home message is that the depth of penetration is related to the tissue characteristics and the frequency of the sound waves. Lower frequency sound waves penetrate deeper into a tissue. The downside is that resolution is related to wavelength, which is the velocity divided by the frequency. The higher resolution of higher frequency comes with a trade-off of greater attenuation and less tissue penetration. The piezo element produces lower voltage levels related to less deformation with reflections from deeper tissue planes. These reflections from deeper planes occur later after the sound pulse generation than do reflections from more superficial tissue. To compensate for the attenuation of sound waves passing through greater amounts of tissue, the gain of an amplifier connected to the piezo element is increased over time after impulse generation. This is called time gain compensation. Modern ophthalmic ultrasonic units have a maximum gain of approximately 90 dB, or 10^9. At this point the noise in the transducer and amplifier are close to the detectable signal, obviating the utility of any increase in gain past this point.

The resolution of an imaging device has two main components, axial resolution and lateral resolution. The better the axial resolution, the greater the ability to separate two closely spaced objects along the path of the beam. Axial resolution is primarily dependent on the wavelength of the probing beam. This distance ideally is approximately ½ of a wavelength for ultrasonography. Lateral resolution is the ability to separate two laterally separated objects. Contact B-scan ultrasonography typically has poor lateral resolution because single piezo transducers produce a relatively broad sound beam. As a consequence, two objects must be laterally separated by a distance large enough to aid detection of their separation by the large diameter probing beam. Because the eye is curved, the wavefront of a broad sound beam also reflects of neighbouring tissues of various depths simultaneously, resulting in lower true axial resolution than what is ideally possible. One solution to this problem is to use an annular phased array of concentric transducers to produce more focused beam characteristics. These probes have the theoretical advantage of both greater lateral resolutions, and because of the narrower beam, greater actual axial resolution in clinical practice. Because of the variables involved, the frequency of ultrasonic transducers used varies with the region being evaluated. To evaluate the globe and anterior orbit, a 10 or 12 MHz probe is commonly used. To evaluate the anterior portions of the eye, a 40 MHz probe can be used. There are weaknesses of ultrasonography. One weakness is there is no indication through independent methods as to where the image was made. The operator has a mental image of the location of the scan, and if landmarks such as the optic nerve are visible and the scan orientation is known, reasonable assumptions can be made as to where the scan was obtained. Otherwise, the person doing the scan may have a good idea about the scan location, but anyone evaluating unlabeled images would be at a loss.

Figures 1 and 2 show clinical examples of using ultrasonography in evaluating the suprachoroidal space in common conditions. Figure 1 shows two patients with vitreous haemorrhage with concurrent suprachoroidal haemorrhages using a 12 MHz concentric phased array probe. Figure 2 shows more anterior imaging ultrasonography using a 40 MHz probe.

Optical Coherence Tomography

The mainstay of imaging the posterior choroid has been OCT. With the advent of EDI and swept-source OCT, the useful imaging range extends to about 1 mm below the surface of the retina. While this is not enough to image the extent of large

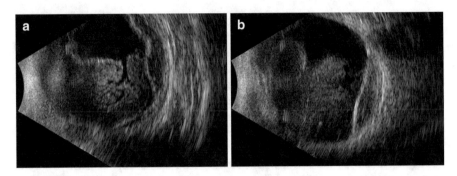

Fig. 1 (**a** and **b**) Two examples of vitreous hemorrhage with hemorrhagic choroidal detachments

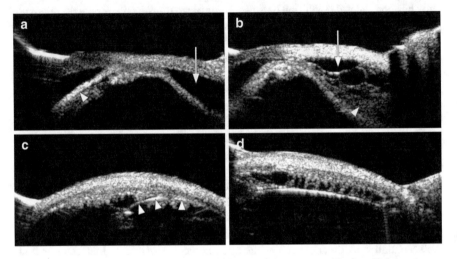

Fig. 2 Anterior segment ultrasonography. (**a**) This eye had a serous ciliochoroidal detachment (arrow). The arrowhead points to the iris. (**b**) There was a resolving hemorrhagic choroidal detachment with pockets of fluid(arrow) and blood (arrowhead). (**c**) This patient had recurrent hemorrhages that were suspected to be from the intraocular lens. Ultrasonography revealed a haptic extended through the ciliary body to the suprachoroidal space (arrowheads). (**d**) This eye had intraocular silicone oil. Although there was nothing wrong with the suprachoroidal space, the ciliary processes are nicely shown, illustrating the resolution of the imaging technique

choroidal detachments, the benefits of OCT include widespread availability, with much higher resolution and repeatability as compared with contact B-scan ultrasonography.

OCT works using the principle of interferometry in which light reflected from the eye is compared with that reflected in a reference arm. The interferogram produced can be evaluated for the strength of reflection as well as the depth from which the reflection arose. The light source used produces short coherence length light. This light is composed of a band of wavelengths. The sum of these wavelengths defines the character of the light. A broad band of wavelengths produce light with a short coherence length. The axial resolution of OCT is essentially equal to the coherence length of the light. In clinical instruments, it is typical to achieve 5–7 μm theoretical resolution. The lateral resolution of OCT is set chiefly by the light source optics and the wavelength of the light. To gain a longer range of imaging OCT instruments use a low numerical aperture. This produces an illuminating beam with a long waist, but the trade-off is the minimal diameter of the beam is relatively large as compared to the axial resolution. As such, the theoretical lateral resolution can be 2–3 times greater than the theoretical axial resolution. The resolution actually achieved in the eye is less than the theoretical resolution because of scatter and optical aberrations including defocus, astigmatism, changing power caused by tear film variations, crystalline lens defects, among many others. Much the same as in ultrasonography, longer wavelengths show greater penetration but less resolution. The range available is large in ultrasonography, from 2 to 100 MHz, while the range in commercial ophthalmic OCT instruments is approximately 25%. Current commercial OCT scanners operate near 100,000 A-scans per second, some more, some less. Acquisition of large, high density images occurs in seconds. These images are shown in the context of an en face image of the eye so that the exact location of the scan is known. OCT instruments with eye tracking can repeat scans over time that are within microns of each other, ensuring accurate comparisons.

The data obtained by OCT (and ultrasonography) is depth resolved and imaging a volume of data can be used to produce 3D renderings. While volume rendering is possible, it is not common with OCT and distinctly less so with ultrasonography of the eye, even though volume rendering is commonly used in ultrasonography of other body structures.

Evaluation of the Choroid and Ambiguities Introduced by the Suprachoroidea

With EDI-OCT and later with swept source OCT, it became possible to evaluate the thickness of the choroid. Early on it was noted that the choroidal thickness measurements could vary, not because of ambiguities about the interface between the RPE and choroid, but what constituted the outer border of the choroid. In many eyes, the choroid does not seem to be bordered directly by the highly reflective sclera. These eyes had an intervening layer or layers between the choroid and the sclera. In publications, this has been termed the suprachoroidal space [12] or the suprachoroidal layer [13] or both [14]. Some confusion may arise in OCT as much as in histologic evaluation. The outer portion of the choroid potentially could be considered to be measured to the outer aspects of the choroidal vascular lumens in the deep choroid. Of course, vessels have walls, which would not be included in this measurement. Other papers have shown measurements to the innermost portion of the suprachoroidal layer [13], which is likely to represent the suprachoroidea. A logical approach would be to follow the histologic convention, which is to include the suprachoroidea as part of the choroid. Therefore, the thickness of the choroid would extend from the outer boundary of the RPE band to the inner portion of the sclera. Given blood vessel, walls of the Haller's layer (large choroidal vessels) may be immediately adjacent to the sclera, and their vessel walls may merge with the scleral reflection, this may still represent a difficulty.

Evaluating the Suprachoroidal Space

Enlargement of the potential space to a real space can occur under a number of conditions. Choroidal effusions are a common consequence of trauma, surgery, inflammation, and drug reactions. This produces hypoechogenic detachments of the peripheral choroid as best seen with ultrasonography for large separations. In the posterior pole, a limited accumulation of fluid has been demonstrated to occur in central serous chorioretinopathy, especially when the subfoveal choroidal thickness exceeds 400 μm [15]. The fluid is hyporeflective, has a polygonal boundary and is not contained by vascular walls. These eyes had a layer of what appeared to be suprachoroidea, and after photodynamic therapy, the choroid thinned, the fluid resolved and the suprachoroidea was not easily visible. This suggests the thickness of the suprachoroidea, or suprachoroidal layer, may be hydrated to varying degrees, which may affect its apparent thickness (Fig. 3).

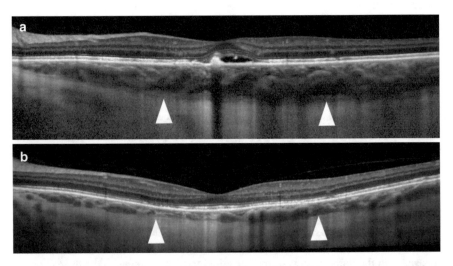

Fig. 3 The outer choroid in central serous chorioretinopathy. (**a**) This patient had central serous chorioretinopathy and had subretinal fluid and loculated fluid in the outer choroid. Note the suprachoroidea, also known as the suprachoroidal layer (arrowheads). (**b**) After the patient had photodynamic therapy, outside of the area contained in this OCT section, the subretinal fluid and choroidal fluid loculations resolved and the suprachoroidea became much thinner (arrowheads). This implies the thickness of the suprachoroidea may vary with hydration

Injection of sodium hyaluronate into the suprachoroidal space has been used to create a temporary buckle for retinal detachment repair [16, 17]. The buckling effect lasts 1–2 weeks, providing time to attain retinal adhesion. Injection of gas into the suprachoroidal space also has the potential to make a buckling effect. As with any suprachoroidal injection, the patient is likely to have pain [18]. However, inadvertent injection of air into the suprachoroidal space during vitrectomy has resulted in death from an air embolism [19].

A similar complementary approach with ultrasonography and OCT can be used to evaluate the suprachoroidal space in the context of drug injections anteriorly or posteriorly using a cannula. It is possible that anterior injections could be monitored in real-time with ultrasonography or anterior segment OCT and posteriorly with either ultrasonography or OCT. These evaluations can be used to help assure the correct location of the cannula and the resultant injection, and also may help in determining the extent of drug dispersion in the suprachoroidal space. Implants into the suprachoroidal space have been proposed as a mechanism of neuromodulation [8]. Although the placement of cannulas, drug injections [20, 21], and devices may be evaluated by ophthalmoscopy, the depth resolution and repeatability of OCT is excellent. In addition, degeneration of choroidal or retinal layers can be determined with OCT but could not be reasonably evaluated by ophthalmoscopy.

Eyes having hypotony after cataract surgery may be suspected to have a cyclodialysis cleft, which provides an alternate drainage mechanism for aqueous to leave the eye via the suprachoroidal space. These may be detected using anterior segment ultrasonography. Glaucoma treatment using cyclodialysis was reported more than a century ago [22], but had a high rate of failure and poor controllability. Superseding cyclodialysis has been the introduction of stents to take fluid from the anterior chamber to the suprachoroidal space [23]. These stents, and the positioning in the suprachoroidal space, have been readily imaged using anterior segment OCT [23]. While the idea behind the stent, the CyPass Micro-Stent, is ingenious, the device was recalled from the market because of endothelial cell loss from the cornea.

Summary

Ultrasonography and OCT are the main methods the suprachoroidal space is evaluated in clinical practice. These methods are flexible and powerful in their present incarnations and are expected to improve in the future. With specific demands created by suprachoroidal therapies, the imaging modalities can be improved to address future needs, as they arise.

References

1. Sohn EH, Khanna A, Tucker BA, et al. Structural and biochemical analyses of choroidal thickness in human donor eyes. Invest Ophthalmol Vis Sci. 2014;55(3):1352–60.

2. Spaide RF, Ledesma-Gil G, Mullins RF. The varying optical coherence tomography appearance of the inner choroid with age: possible explanation and histologic correlate. Retina. 2021;41(5):1071–5.
3. Trier K, Olsen EB, Ammitzbøll T. Regional glycosaminoglycans composition of the human sclera. Acta Ophthalmol. 1990;68(3):304–6.
4. Hogan MJ, Alvarado JA, Weddell JE. Histology of the human eye. In: An atlas and textbook. Philadelphia, PA: W.B. Saunders Company; 1971.
5. Rai Udo J, Young SA, Thrimawithana TR, et al. The suprachoroidal pathway: a new drug delivery route to the back of the eye. Drug Discov Today. 2015;20(4):491–5.
6. Chen M, Li X, Liu J, Han Y, Cheng L. Safety and pharmacodynamics of suprachoroidal injection of triamcinolone acetonide as a controlled ocular drug release model. J Control Release. 2015;203:109–17.
7. Olsen TW, Feng X, Wabner K, et al. Cannulation of the suprachoroidal space: a novel drug delivery methodology to the posterior segment. Am J Ophthalmol. 2006;142(5):777–87.
8. Bareket L, Barriga-Rivera A, Zapf MP, Lovell NH, Suaning GJ. Progress in artificial vision through suprachoroidal retinal implants. J Neural Eng. 2017;14(4):045002.
9. Kim SH, Galbán CJ, Lutz RJ, et al. Assessment of subconjunctival and intrascleral drug delivery to the posterior segment using dynamic contrast-enhanced magnetic resonance imaging. Invest Ophthalmol Vis Sci. 2007;48(2):808–14.
10. Gunenc U, Maden A, Kaynak S, Pirnar T. Magnetic resonance imaging and computed tomography in the detection and localisation of intraocular foreign bodies. Doc Ophthalmol. 1992;81(4):369–78.
11. Li SK, Lizak MJ, Jeong EK. MRI in ocular drug delivery. NMR Biomed. 2008;21(9):941–56.
12. Rahman W, Chen FK, Yeoh J, et al. Repeatability of manual subfoveal choroidal thickness measurements in healthy subjects using the technique of enhanced depth imaging optical coherence tomography. Invest Ophthalmol Vis Sci. 2011;52(5):2267–71.
13. Yiu G, Pecen P, Sarin N, et al. Characterisation of the choroid-scleral junction and suprachoroidal layer in healthy individuals on enhanced-depth imaging optical coherence tomography. JAMA Ophthalmol. 2014;132(2):174–81.
14. Michalewska Z, Michalewski J, Nawrocka Z, et al. Suprachoroidal layer and suprachoroidal space delineating the outer margin of the choroid in swept-source optical coherence tomography. Retina. 2015;35(2):244–9.
15. Spaide RF, Ryan EH Jr. Loculation of fluid in the posterior choroid in eyes with central serous chorioretinopathy. Am J Ophthalmol. 2015;160(6):1211–6.
16. Poole TA, Sudarsky RD. Suprachoroidal implantation for the treatment of retinal detachment. Ophthalmology. 1986;93(11):1408–12.
17. Mittl RN, Tiwari R. Suprachoroidal injection of sodium hyaluronate as an 'internal' buckling procedure. Ophthalmic Res. 1987;19(5):255–60.
18. Jabaly-Habib HY, Fineberg EM, Tornambe PE, et al. Prolonged pain following unintentional injection of gas into the suprachoroidal space during pneumatic retinopexy. Retina. 2003;23(5):722–3.
19. Morris RE, Sapp MR, Oltmanns MH, Kuhn F. Presumed air by vitrectomy embolisation (PAVE) a potentially fatal syndrome. Br J Ophthalmol. 2014;98(6):765–8.
20. Patel SR, Lin AS, Edelhauser HF, Prausnitz MR. Suprachoroidal drug delivery to the back of the eye using hollow microneedles. Pharm Res. 2011;28(1):166–76.
21. Patel SR, Berezovsky DE, McCarey BE, Zarnitsyn V, Edelhauser HF, Prausnitz MR. Targeted administration into the suprachoroidal space using a microneedle for drug delivery to the posterior segment of the eye. Invest Ophthalmol Vis Sci. 2012;53(8):4433–41.
22. Heine L. Die Cyclodialyse, eine neue glaukomoperation. Dtsch Med Wochenschr. 1905;31(21):824–6.
23. Saheb H, Ianchulev T, Ahmed II. Optical coherence tomography of the suprachoroid after CyPass micro-stent implantation for the treatment of open-angle glaucoma. Br J Ophthalmol. 2014;98(1):19–23.

Suprachoroidal Haemorrhage

Thomas H. Williamson, Aman Chandra, and Mahmut Dogramaci

Introduction

Suprachoroidal haemorrhage (SCH) is relatively uncommon, surprisingly so given the highly vascular structure of the choroid. Possible mechanisms for the rupture of blood vessels causing haemorrhage are hypotony, distortion of vascular architecture and direct injury to the blood vessels. Arterioles, venules, and capillaries are all potential sources of bleeding. More sudden and severe bleeds are attributed to the arterioles rather than the venules but evidence for this is not strong. The haemorrhage preferentially collects in the suprachoroidal space and with relatively little resistance from surrounding tissues may fill a large proportion of the vitreous cavity. The thrombus formed as a result can contain 3–4 ml of blood, and therefore is slow to clear. This is in keeping with other large haemorrhages seen elsewhere in the body, e.g. deep vein thrombosis or sub-epidural bleeds.

Pathogenesis

Some SCH may result from rupture of ciliary arteries in the suprachoroidal space. Long posterior ciliary arteries pierce the posterior part of the sclera near the optic nerve, and run forward between the sclera and choroid, to the ciliary muscle, where

T. H. Williamson (✉)
Department of Ophthalmology, St. Thomas' Hospital, London, UK
e-mail: tom@retinasurgery.co.uk

A. Chandra
Southend University Hospital, Southend, UK

M. Dogramaci
The Princess Alexandra Hospital, Harlow, UK

they divide into branches. Suprachoroidal haemorrhages are usually observed at or anterior to the equator. A histopathologic study of an eye with an expulsive SCH has shown a ruptured artery and a haemorrhage that spread anteriorly as far as scleral spur leading to forward rotation of the ciliary body [1].

Dynamics of Suprachoroidal Haemorrhage

To understand the dynamics of suprachoroidal vessel rupture, it is worth explaining the process in 2 phases. Phase 1 covers the factors that lead to ciliary artery rupture and phase 2 covers the factors that govern dissemination of blood in extravascular space.

Phase 1: Ciliary Artery Rupture

Ciliary arteries like any other tubular structure are exposed to two different forms of strain. The first is inflation related strain and the second is elongation related strain. Inflation related strain occurs when the intra-tubular pressure exceeds the extra-tubular pressure, which can be due to an increased intratubular pressure (e.g. systemic hypertension) or a relative drop in extra-tubular pressure (e.g. ocular hypotony) or a combination of both. Elongation related strain occurs when the tubular structure is stretched in one direction. In both cases, the strains lead to increased levels of stress in the wall of the tubular structure leading to failure and extravasation at its weakest location. One analogy is a hose attached to a tap: an increase in stress levels in the hose can result in its detachment from the tap. Stress levels in the hose can rise if the hose is over inflated because of a blockage in the line and also when it is pulled away from the tap.

Finite element analysis (FEA) shows that a 30% increase in the pressure at the arteriolar end of a capillary, or reducing the intraocular pressure to 0 mmHg, both independently increase the shear stress in the capillary blood vessels by one- to twofold. Mechanically stretching the capillaries by 4% results in a 43-fold increase in shear stress on the capillary wall. This emphasizes the role of globe distortion during surgery in developing suprachoroidal haemorrhage (Fig. 1).

It is useful to think about the eye as a fragile tissue that can break or tear if not handled carefully during an operation. Therefore, it is important to minimise distortion of the globe. Take care when indenting and tightening sutures over an external buckle and maintain intraocular pressure during the entire duration of surgery.

Phase 2: Dissemination of Blood into the Extravascular Space

Rupture of the ciliary artery leads to extravasation of blood from the artery into the choroid. Within the choroid, resistance to the expansion is generated from surrounding intact vasculature, from the outer layers of the eye wall, mainly the sclera, from

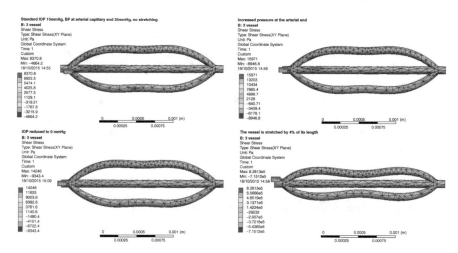

Fig. 1 Finite element analysis of shear stress in the capillary wall. Upper left: shows shear stress at the capillary vessels with intra luminal pressure of 35 mmHg and intra-ocular pressure of 15 mmHg. Upper right: shows shear stress at the capillary vessels with intra luminal pressure of 46 mmHg and intra-ocular pressure of 15 mmHg. Lower left: shows shear stress at the capillary vessels with intra luminal pressure of 35 mmHg and intra-ocular pressure of zero. Lower right: shows shear stress at the capillary vessels with intra luminal pressure of 35 mmHg and intra-ocular pressure of 15 mmHg being stretched by 4% of its horizontal length

the inner layers of the eye wall, mainly Bruch's membrane, and from scattered focal and linear adhesions between the different layers of the eye wall.

Bruch's Membrane and Sclera

Both Bruch' membrane and the sclera have high stiffness compared to other layers of the eye wall; therefore, they resist deformation. In fact, Bruch's membrane may be up to 3 times stiffer than the sclera itself. Young's modulus for sclera is 5.5 MPa and for Bruch's membrane it can be as high as 18.8 MPa in elderly patients [2, 3]. However, higher stiffness of tissue does not necessarily mean better protection against expansion, because the thickness of the tissue is also important. The sclera is approximately one hundred times thicker than Bruch's membrane, with average scleral thickness at the equator of 420μm, compared to the thickness of Bruch's membrane which is only 2–4μm [4, 5]. Because of this difference in thickness, when a suprachoroidal haemorrhage puts an equal amount of pressure both on the sclera and Bruch's membrane, the stress level in Bruch's membrane increases by approximately 15,000 times more than that in the sclera and therefore it deforms more than the sclera. When the stress level in Bruch's membrane exceeds its yield stress threshold, it ruptures, leading to the extravasation of blood. Layers that are too thin or do not have significantly different material properties are usually ignored in modelling, as this approach makes the modelling more memory efficient for computer processors. It is also worth noting that although pressure gradients on either side of the ocular wall layers contribute to the spread of suprachoroidal haemorrhage, such effects are not included in our modelling to improve computing efficiencies (Figs. 2 and 3).

In exceptional circumstances, when the sclera is too thin as in myopic patients, some deformation could also happen in the sclera early on during the process, this may allow more space for the expansion of the haemorrhage and minimising the deformation and stress in Bruch's membrane (Fig. 4).

Scattered Focal Adhesions Between Eye Wall Layers

Focal attachment between the layers of the eye wall, at the ampullae of the vortex veins and the arteries as they cross the SCS, anchor the layers to each other leading to a "cushioned upholstery" effect on the suprachoroidal haemorrhage. Although this kind of adhesion provides protection against free expansion of suprachoroidal haemorrhage into the vitreous cavity, it can also redirect the expansion, leading to circumferential spread of the haemorrhage. This could be missed by an unwary surgeon, who might underestimate the size of the haemorrhage. (Fig. 5) It is therefore important to carefully check all quadrants for circumferential expansion once a localised suprachoroidal haemorrhage is detected.

Linear Adhesions at Ora Serrata

Linear borders of the suprachoroidal space at the scleral spur tend to barricade the haemorrhage stopping the anterior expansion of the suprachoroidal swelling (Fig. 6) and leading to increase in the height of the suprachoroidal swelling posteriorly.

Clinical Presentation

Aetiology
- Trauma
- The different categories of injury as per the Birmingham Eye Trauma Terminology (BETT) [6, 7] are all associated with potential for SCH. However, it is penetrating injury and scleral rupture which are most associated with this complication. Severe disruption of the interior structures of the eye are seen, often with accompanying anterior segment injury and retinal detachment with an extremely high rate of formation of proliferative vitreo-retinopathy (PVR). (Fig. 7)

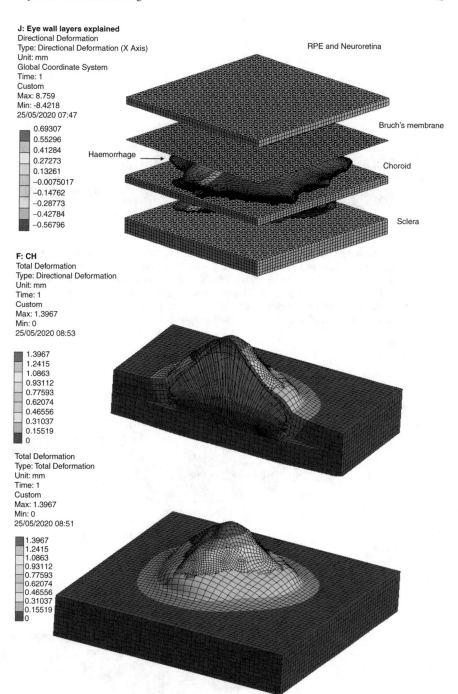

Fig. 2 Comparison of the thickness of the layers of the eye wall. Top: From top downward the retina (200μ), Bruch's membrane (2 microns), the choroid (200μ) and the sclera (420μ). The irregular area at the centre of the choroid represents suprachoroidal haemorrhage. The distance between the layers are exaggerated for demonstration purposes. Middle: shows FEA of choroidal haemorrhage with retinal layers at their normal distance from each other. Bottom: shows a cross section for FEA of choroidal haemorrhage with retinal layers at their normal distance from each other

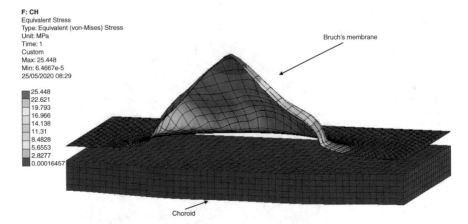

Fig. 3 Finite element analysis of suprachoroidal haemorrhage. Because of the difference in thickness of Bruch's membrane and the sclera, when a suprachoroidal haemorrhage puts an equal amount of pressure both on the sclera and Bruch's membrane, the stress level in Bruch's membrane increases by 15,000 times in the sclera and therefore Bruch's membrane deforms more than the sclera. When the stress level in Bruch's membrane exceeds its yields stress threshold, it ruptures leading to the extravasation of blood into the subretinal space

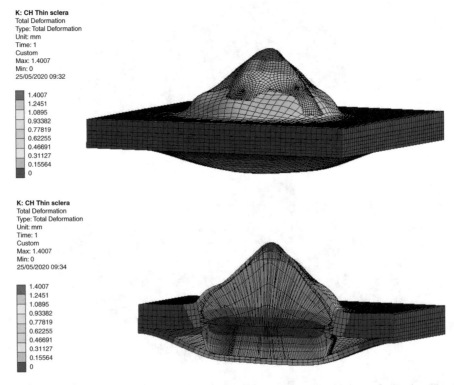

Fig. 4 Finite element analysis of suprachoroidal haemorrhage with 50% thinner sclera. Top: scleral bulge is visible inferiorly. Such a bulge is likely to reduce the stress in Bruch's membrane and result in less deformation and smaller height of suprachoroidal haemorrhage within vitreous cavity. Bottom: shows a cross section of the same analysis above

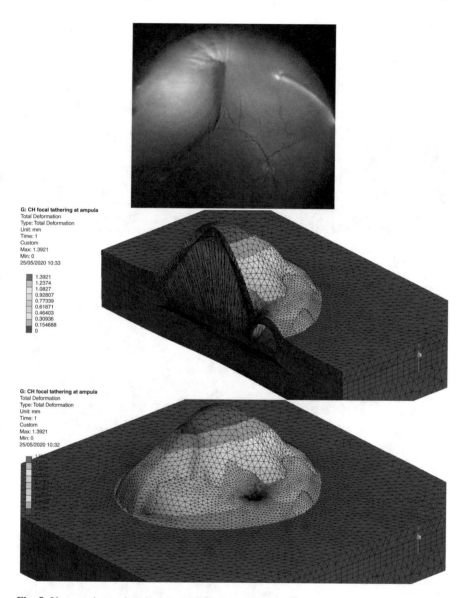

Fig. 5 Vortex veins anchor the layers of the eye wall to each other, giving a "cushioned uphol-stery" effect to the suprachoroidal haemorrhage (top image). Such attachments provide protection against free expansion of suprachoroidal haemorrhages into the vitreous cavity and redirect the expansion leading to the circumferential spread (middle and bottom images)

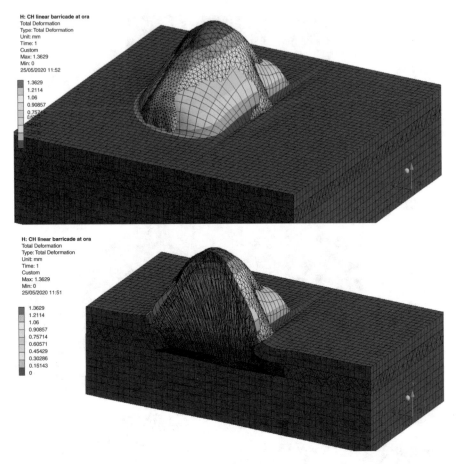

Fig. 6 Linear adhesions at the ora serrata can lead to increased height of the suprachoroidal swelling

Fig. 7 This suprachoroidal haemorrhage is so severe that it has pushed the choroid and retina up behind the lens

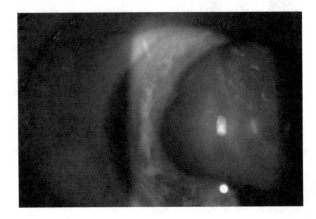

- Surgery

  - Massive SCH is a rare risk of anterior segment surgery and can be seen late as an expulsive haemorrhage [8–13]. An incidence of 0.04% has been described in the UK [14, 15]. The delay in detection peroperatively results in a large and often catastrophic haemorrhage (Fig. 8). This is a rare risk during surgery such as cataract extraction [14], trabeculectomy [16, 17], glaucoma drainage implants [18]) and corneal grafting [9, 11, 19–22]. Wound leakage or insufficient infusion result in hypotony which allows vessel rupture in at risk individuals with arteriopathy, high myopia or hypertension. Bleeds are made worse by delayed thrombus formation in those on anti-thrombotic or anti-platelet agents. The haemorrhage may occur intra-operatively or be delayed and occur after surgery [17, 18, 23–29]. (Fig. 9)
  - A late SCH can be seen in glaucoma for example when needling of a trabecular flap is performed [30].
  - Severe haemorrhage occurs in 0.14–0.17% of pars plana vitrectomy (PPV) but smaller self-limiting haemorrhages which resolve spontaneously may occur [31–38]. In vitreoretinal surgery SCH is associated with the application of a scleral explant [35] [38] or as a result of intraocular hypotony. The former distorts blood vessels risking rupture and bleeds. The latter may be due to a mismatch between intraocular and infusion pressures, especially if vacuum is

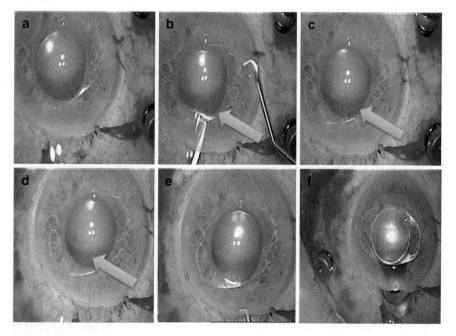

Fig. 8 Suprachoroidal haemorrhage developing over 1 min during iris clip IOL Insertion. (**a**) IOL in place, due to enclave final haptic; (**b**) Early SCH noted (arrow); (**c** and **d**) SCH growing (arrow); (**e**) No Red reflex; (**f**) Prolapse of iris

Fig. 9 A suprachoroidal haemorrhage is settling after a complicated cataract operation. Secondary retinal detachment can occur with PVR. Close observation is required

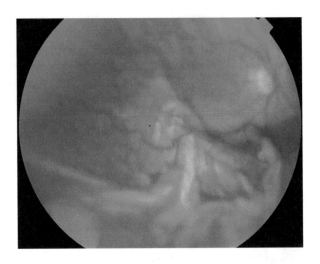

created with continuous aspiration. This may be less common with small gauge systems, and vitrectomy systems which attempt to match infusion and vacuum. Tilting eyes during surgery may kink infusion lines and result in sudden reduction in infusion pressure. Finally, as infusion lines in small gauge PPV are not sutured, they can become misplaced. This may result in detachment of the infusion from the trochar giving hypotony. Misdirection of the trochar in the eye may lead to suprachoroidal infusion and secondary rupture of choroidal vessels. (Fig. 10)

SCH during PPV tends to be more localised partly due to earlier recognition and better intraocular pressure control than in anterior segment surgery.

- Spontaneous

    - Highly myopic eyes have occasionally been described with a spontaneous presentation of SCH [39]. The thin sclera of these eye seems to allow more rapid resolution of SCH. SCH has been described particularly in those patients on systemic antithrombotic therapy [40, 41].

- Systemic conditions

    - Malignant hypertension may be a precursor to SCH [42].

Risk factors:
- Arteriopathy
- High myopia
- Hypertension
- Antiplatelet and antithrombotic drugs

    - These have not been found to increase rates of SCH in cataract surgery [43] and warfarin has not been shown to increase the risk in vitrectomy [32].

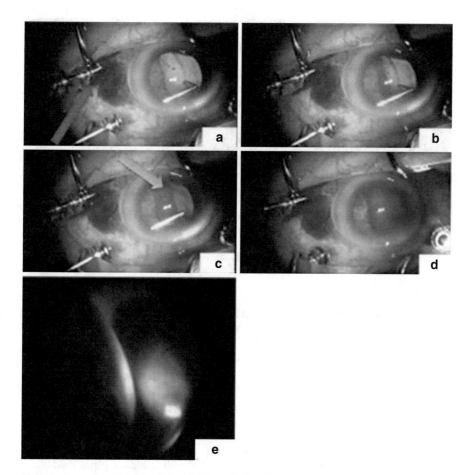

Fig. 10 Suprachoroidal infusion. (**a**) Note displaced infusion line (red arrow); (**b** and **c**) Suprachoroidal infusion developing over 3 s (blue arrow); (**d**) Loss of red reflex; (**e**) Posterior segment view (massive suprachoroidal infusion)

However, they may be associated with increased severity of the haemorrhage. The effect of antiplatelet medication is likely to be more relevant in microsurgery than anticoagulants, although neither have been demonstrated convincingly to be important in the risk of developing SCH.

Symptoms
- Reduced vision
- Visual loss depends on the location and extent of the SCH. Most are situated in the peripheral posterior segment. If the SCH is localised, vision may be good (Fig. 11). More severe SCH will reduce vision as the elevation blocks the macula. SCH in the macula itself is a bad prognostic sign for recovery of vision.

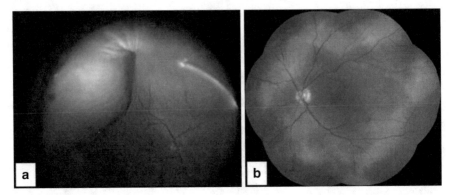

Fig. 11 Suprachoroidal haemorrhage and resolution. (**a**) Suprachoroidal haemorrhage after cataract surgery complicated with dropped nuclear lens fragment. Notice the dome shape, and dark hue to the elevated areas. The haemorrhage was drained, and fortunately the macula was not involved. (**b**) As the macula was uninvolved, the visual outcome was excellent

- Pain

    - In severe cases with high elevation there is a severe aching pain. This subsides in time (1 month) even if the elevation persists.
    - Pain occurs possibly from stretch of ciliary nerves or from significant intraocular hypertension if the SCH is exceptionally large.

- Visual field loss

    - The peripheral position of most SCH restricts visual fields in these eyes.

Clinical signs on examination
- Dark red/greenish smooth elevation
- The elevation has a deep red/black or a greenish colouration in pigmented fundi. The surface is smooth or wrinkled.
- Immobile

    - Unlike neuroretinal elevations (such as RRD) the tissue is not mobile.

- Peripheral

    - The location of SCH is primarily in the fundal periphery spreading from there towards the macula.(Figs. 12 and 13)

- Macula

    - Often the macula is spared though subretinal blood may gravitate there. If the macula is involved in the SCH there is poor prognosis for visual recovery.

- Tethered at the optic nerve head

    - In eyes with a poor fundal view an ultrasound will show the elevation limited posteriorly at the optic disc margin.

Fig. 12 A diffuse area of shallow choroidal haemorrhage is shown superiorly in a high myope. The haemorrhages although occur more commonly in high myopes often clear quickly in these eyes

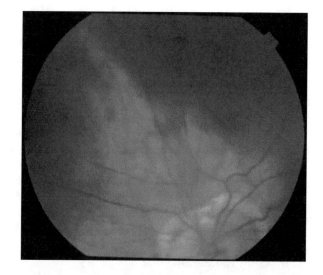

Fig. 13 A suprachoroidal haemorrhage from PPV and inferior scleral buckle. The eye has been filled with non-compressible silicone oil to try to limit the spread of the haemorrhage

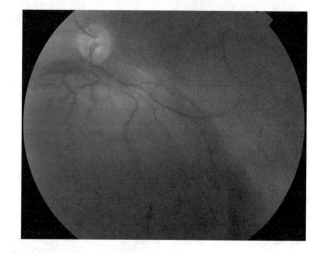

- Complete or subtotal SCH may occur with "kissing choroidals" where the opposing elevations are in contact with each other centrally. Macula is usually but not always involved in such cases.

Fundal characteristics
- Dome shaped choroidal elevation due to solid clot
    - Partial
    - Subtotal
    - Total (or complete)
- Associated intraocular haemorrhage

It is unusual for the SCH not to leak into other layers of the eye with further consequences for secondary complications and haemorrhage in other layers.

- Subretinal space
- Vitreous cavity
- Anterior chamber (hyphaema)

Complications

- Retinal detachment with PVR

    - RD is a common secondary effect. It can be rhegmatogenous (formation of a break with rapid loss of tissues and vitreous traction in an open eye) or tractional (with appositional SCH). RD and SCH are an unfavourable combination, PVR ensues rapidly and severely. This is particularly an issue with appositional SCH such as is seen in "kissing choroidals". It is worth considering an early intervention in such cases to reduce the risk of PVR development. (Fig. 14)

- Hypotony and phthisis bulbi

    - The SCH may affect the function of the ciliary body either with ciliary body detachment or fibrosis. This may contribute to a risk of hypotony in these eyes in addition to the underlying cause of the SCH.

- Hyphaema and corneal staining

    - SCH will leak blood, and some will enter the anterior chamber. It is important to monitor intraocular pressure with hyphaema due to the risk of glaucoma and corneal staining. (Fig. 15)

- Retinal toxicity

    Subretinal blood and multi-layered haemorrhage is likely to be toxic to the photoreceptors, demonstrated by poor visual outcome with sub macular SCH.

- Mechanical barrier

Fig. 14 Ultrasound B scan demonstrating "kissing choroidals"(arrows) due to suprachoroidal haemorrhage secondary to complicated cataract surgery

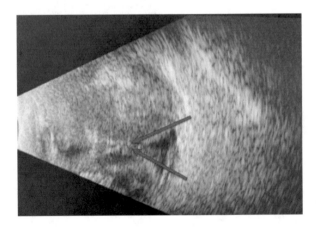

Fig. 15 Subtotal
hyphaema post massive
suprachoroidal
haemorrhage during
complicated anterior
segment surgery with late
recognition

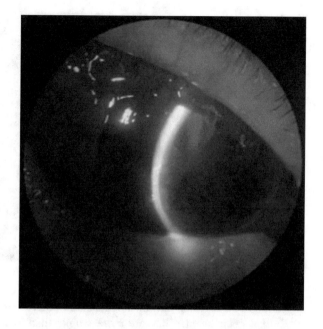

- Suprachoroidal blood may impair normal metabolism of the choroid and outer retina
- Blood can lead to formation of chorioretinal fibrosis especially if traumatic
- Macular detachment with haemorrhage (Submacular haemorrhage)

Investigation: Ultrasound

This is a key investigation. Often visualisation of the posterior segment is reduced due to anterior segment pathology or vitreous opacity. Ultrasound is required to identify the layers of the eye and assess the severity of the SCH. In addition, the macula should be assessed for elevation. Serial scans are required to detect resolution of the SCH and for the determination of the need to perform surgery (Figs. 16, 17, and 18).

Differential diagnosis
- Choroidal effusion: Effusion tends to have a clearer appearance on clinical examination. Ultrasonography demonstrates a more echo lucent (dark) appearance than haemorrhage.
- Malignant melanoma (MM). Clinically, melanoma may have lipofuscin deposits at the level of the RPE. MM tend to be dome or mushroom shaped. Ultrasonography may help differentiate between MM and small SCH. MM tend to have medium to low internal reflectivity. They may also have an acoustically silent zone within

Fig. 16 B-scan Ultrasound
reveals a localised elevated
choroidal lesion clinically
diagnosed as choroidal
haemorrhage which can be
measured

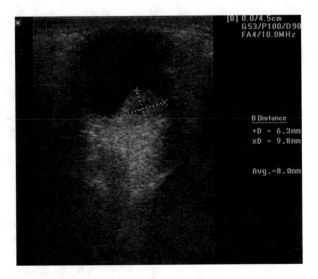

the lesion and overlying choroidal excavation and orbital shadowing. A short
period of observation may also demonstrate regression of small SCH.

- Retinal detachment: They are more mobile than SCH or choroidal effusions.
  This can be demonstrated clinically and by ultrasonography. Retinal detachments do not tend to conform to the "dome" shape of SCH.

Management of SCH

Suggestions for avoiding SCH during surgery:

1. Be particularly vigilant of patients who may be at risk of SCH (high myopes,
   patients who have had a previous SCH, arteriopathic status)
2. Maintain constant IOP during surgery and avoid ocular hypotony

   - Self-sealing wounds [2]
   - Remember the basic microsurgical principle of pivoting instruments at the
     wound, to minimise egress of intraocular fluid
   - Surgical systems with IOP control

3. Minimise inflammation stimulating procedures, such as contact with the iris
4. Adequate infusion pressures

   - Be aware, when using systems with passive infusion, an increase in the height
     of the operating table must be compensated by an increase in the height of the
     infusion bottle

5. Minimise distortion to the globe and underlying choroidal vasculature

   - Gentle indentation to minimise a blood vessel injury
   - Tightening sutures over an external ocular device with minimal disturbance to
     the ocular anatomy and choroidal vasculature

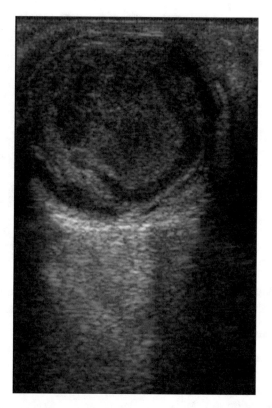

Fig. 17 A suprachoroidal haemorrhage develops into a catastrophic haemorrhage because the cataract surgeon does not notice the SCH until it is too late. The surgeon performing vitrectomy usually notices early signs of SCH under direct visualisation and therefore can react more quickly to limit the size of the haemorrhage. In this patient an expulsive SCH occurred during an extracapsular cataract extraction. At 3 weeks there was haemolysis and partial resolution of the haemorrhage allowing space to perform surgery. Using an anterior chamber maintainer, the vitreous haemorrhage was removed and liquified choroidal haemorrhage expelled. The eye was filled with silicone oil to await further choroidal haemorrhage resolution and repeat surgery

- Avoid deep scleral sutures
- Insert perfluorocarbon liquids to stabilise the posterior segment in vitrectomised eyes to prevent distortion of the globe during complex anterior segment surgery [44].

6. Check the IOP at the end of the operation and aim to leave the eye firm at the end of the procedure.

- Secure the wound if it is leaking.
- If necessary, inject saline through a paracentesis into the anterior chamber in a fluid filled eye, watch for posterior movement of the lens iris diaphragm in a gas filled eye, use a 30G needle on the gas syringe to top up gas through the pars plana.
- Note that the IOP will drop after removal of the lid speculum. The speculum is acting to increase the orbital pressure and therefore the IOP. Therefore, a

Fig. 18 An ultrasound of an eye with choroidal haemorrhage from trauma

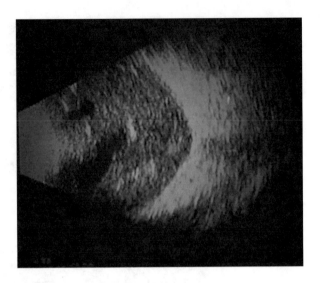

soft eye before the speculum is removed can become incredibly soft after it is removed. It is safer to have a very firm eye prior to removing the speculum.

Important considerations when choroidal haemorrhage arises

1. Stop leakage and maintain IOP.
2. Raise the pressure in the globe.
3. Allow time for a clot to form.
4. Finish the operation and close.
5. If tamponade is required, a liquid is better than a gas as the former is non-compressible.

What to do if choroidal haemorrhage occurs during anterior segment surgery

1. Early recognition: If there is a sudden change in IOP, consider whether SCH has developed. Sudden changes can occur during any moment, but particularly if a complication such as posterior capsular rupture develops. Subsequent hardening/increase in IOP must alert the surgeon to the possibility of SCH.
2. When recognised, close the main wound as efficiently as possible. Replace any expelled intraocular tissue if possible, but not at the expense of closing the wound.

What to do if choroidal haemorrhage occurs during posterior segment surgery

- Raise the infusion bottle height to 60 cm or pressurised system to 40–50 mmHg.
- Allow time for a clot to form over the leaking blood vessel before dropping the IOP by removing an instrument, at least 1 min (count to sixty slowly or watch the clock). Do not be tempted to do anything else until you have given a chance for the clot on the ruptured blood vessel to plug the hole in the vessel wall.

- If there is only a small haemorrhage at the end of the operation, finish the operation and close.
- It is best to avoid leaving the eye gas filled because gas is compressible and will allow postoperative enlargement of the haemorrhage. If tamponade is required, you should use silicone oil which is non compressible.
- If there is significant haemorrhage during vitrectomy ask the assistant to prepare silicone oil for infusion, keep the instruments in the eye and have the assistant attach the oil to the three way tap on the infusion. Start the oil pump, switch to a flute needle, and fill the eye with oil.

Note, we suspect that choroidal haemorrhages are so catastrophic in anterior segment surgery because the surgeon sees the haemorrhage late i.e. when the red reflex starts to change. This is not the case in vitreoretinal surgery when the haemorrhage is seen early and can be controlled as above. Therefore, small haemorrhages are recognised; suggesting a higher "rate" of choroidal haemorrhage than anterior segment surgery, which is likely to represent recognition bias. Nevertheless, these SCH can be kept small and resolve with less morbidity.

The key is to allow the blood clot to form to plug the hole in the blood vessel.

Subsequent management of SCH
- Observation
- Monitor IOP
- Watch for RRD and PVR
- Surgical drainage methods

Small SCH may be observed, particularly if the macula is unaffected. Slow resolution is likely to occur, particularly in SCH which may have a serous element (just as post trabeculectomy SCH or spontaneous myopic SCH).

If the macula is involved, or kissing choroidal haemorrhage is present, intervention is likely to reduce visual morbidity.

In these cases, an initial period of observation is a prudent approach.

This is to allow thrombolysis of the SCH and closure of the rupture in the blood vessel wall by healing. Thrombolysis of whole blood takes up to 20 h. Larger bleeds can be much slower [45]. Animal models of liquefaction of thrombi in the suprachoroidal space suggest that 1–2 weeks are necessary for this to occur [46]. The dilemma posed is that evacuating too early may result in a repeat rupture of the blood vessel rupture. Too long a wait may lead to fibrotic organisation and solidification of the SCH.

Therefore, although small series of earlier intervention are reported [47], most reports suggest a short delay [27, 48].

To aid liquefaction, there are reports of suprachoroidal injection of recombinant tissue plasminogen activator (rTPA) prior to drainage [49]. An example of its use allowing drainage 3 days after massive SCH post complicated extracapsular extraction, is shown in Fig. 19.

The technique recommended for SCH drainage involves placement of an anterior chamber infusion (in phakic or pseudophakic eyes). An incision is then made posteriorly, to enter the SCH, but avoiding the vortex veins (Fig. 19). Increasing the intraocular pressure with digital pressure and manoeuvering of the eye may allow further expulsion of SCH.

When combined with pars plana vitrectomy, there are techniques suggesting use of valve less trocars inserted transsclerally and into the suprachoroidal space to aid drainage [50]. It is recommendable to use non compressible tamponades such as saline or silicone oil, rather than intraocular gas. Only use the last, if confident that the SCH is unlikely to extend. Finally, short term perfluorocarbon liquid may be left in situ to aid continued drainage. Sclerotomy sites do not need to be sutured.

When operating on an eye with previous resolved SCH use extra methods to control IOP and choroidal stability. For example, perfluorocarbon liquids can be inserted into the vitreous cavity of vitrectomised eyes to prevent rupture of choroidal vessels during anterior segment surgery [44]. (Fig. 20).

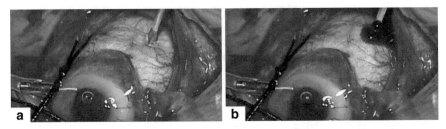

Fig. 19 Drainage of suprachoroidal haemorrhage. (**a**) Incision with 20G blade 8–10 mm posterior to limbus. (**b**) Expulsion of suprachoroidal haemorrhage with aid of positive pressure of anterior infusion

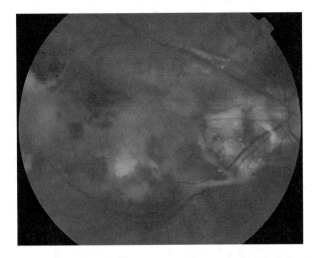

Fig. 20 Complications with the infusion cannula can be catastrophic. A danger is movement of the tip of the cannula into the subretinal or suprachoroidal space during perioperative hypotony. In this case this caused insertion of suprachoroidal air during air exchange with secondary haemorrhage in the macula. An AC infusion was inserted, and the air was removed via a sclerotomy. The posterior chamber infusion was repositioned. The macular haemorrhage was only partially removed via retinotomy probably because there was some blood in the suprachoroidal space. A postoperative image is shown, silicone oil was inserted

References

1. Wolter JR. Expulsive hemorrhage: a study of histopathological details. Graefes Arch Clin Exp Ophthalmol. 1982;219(4):155–8.
2. Williamson TH. Intraocular surgery, a basic surgical guide. Berlin: Springer; 2016.
3. Chan W, Hussain A, Marshall J. Youngs modulus of Bruchs membrane: implications for AMD. Investig Ophthalmol Vis Sci. 2007;48(13):2187.
4. Lee CJ, Vroom JA, Fishman HA, Bent SF. Determination of human lens capsule permeability and its feasibility as a replacement for Bruch's membrane. Biomaterials. 2006;27(8):1670–8.
5. Vurgese S, Panda-Jonas S, Jonas JB. Scleral thickness in human eyes. PLoS One. 2012;7(1):e29692.
6. Kuhn F, Maisiak R, Mann L, Mester V, Morris R, Witherspoon CD. The ocular trauma score (OTS). Ophthalmol Clin N Am. 2002;15(2):163–5. vi
7. Kuhn F, Morris R, Witherspoon CD, Heimann K, Jeffers JB, Treister G. A standardized classification of ocular trauma. Ophthalmology. 1996;103(2):240–3.
8. Obuchowska I, Mariak Z. Risk factors of massive suprachoroidal hemorrhage during extracapsular cataract extraction surgery. Eur J Ophthalmol. 2005;15(6):712–7. https://doi.org/10.1177/112067210501500609.
9. Reynolds MG, Haimovici R, Flynn HW Jr, DiBernardo C, Byrne SF, Feuer W. Suprachoroidal hemorrhage. Clinical features and results of secondary surgical management. Ophthalmology. 1993;100(4):460–5.
10. Sharma T, Virdi DS, Parikh S, Gopal L, Badrinath SS, Mukesh BN. A case-control study of suprachoroidal hemorrhage during pars plana vitrectomy. Ophthalmic Surg Lasers. 1997;28(8):640–4.
11. Speaker MG, Guerriero PN, Met JA, Coad CT, Berger A, Marmor M. A case-control study of risk factors for intraoperative suprachoroidal expulsive hemorrhage. Ophthalmology. 1991;98(2):202–9.
12. Welch JC, Spaeth GL, Benson WE. Massive suprachoroidal hemorrhage. Follow-up and outcome of 30 cases. Ophthalmology. 1988;95(9):1202–6.
13. Wong KK, Saleh TA, Gray RH. Suprachoroidal hemorrhage during cataract surgery in a vitrectomized eye. J Cataract Refract Surg. 2005;31(6):1242–3. https://doi.org/10.1016/j.jcrs.2004.10.073.
14. Ling R, Cole M, James C, Kamalarajah S, Foot B, Shaw S. Suprachoroidal haemorrhage complicating cataract surgery in the UK: epidemiology, clinical features, management, and outcomes. Br J Ophthalmol. 2004;88(4):478–80.
15. Ling R, Kamalarajah S, Cole M, James C, Shaw S. Suprachoroidal haemorrhage complicating cataract surgery in the UK: a case control study of risk factors. Br J Ophthalmol. 2004;88(4):474–7. https://doi.org/10.1136/bjo.2003.026179.
16. Hussain N, Hussain A, Khan NA. Favorable outcome after choroidal drainage for postoperative kissing suprachoroidal hemorrhage following trabeculectomy in a high myopic vitrectomised eye. Saudi J Ophthalmol. 2018;32(2):146–50. https://doi.org/10.1016/j.sjopt.2017.10.002.
17. Lin HZ, Huang CT, Lee YC. A blood clot hanging in the anterior chamber due to delayed suprachoroidal hemorrhage after trabeculectomy. Ci Ji Yi Xue Za Zhi. 2016;28(2):73–5. https://doi.org/10.1016/j.tcmj.2015.06.003.
18. Balekudaru S, Basu T, Sen P, Bhende P, Lingam V, George R. Risk factors and outcomes of management of delayed suprachoroidal haemorrhage following Ahmed glaucoma valve implantation in children. Br J Ophthalmol. 2020;104(1):115–20. https://doi.org/10.1136/bjophthalmol-2018-313804.
19. Bandivadekar P, Gupta S, Sharma N. Intraoperative suprachoroidal hemorrhage after penetrating keratoplasty: case series and review of literature. Eye Contact Lens. 2016;42(3):206–10. https://doi.org/10.1097/ICL.0000000000000164.
20. Dockery PW, Joubert K, Parker JS, Parker JS. Suprachoroidal hemorrhage during Descemet membrane endothelial keratoplasty. Cornea. 2020;39(3):376–8. https://doi.org/10.1097/ICO.0000000000002199.

21. Ingraham HJ, Donnenfeld ED, Perry HD. Massive suprachoroidal hemorrhage in penetrating keratoplasty. Am J Ophthalmol. 1989;108(6):670–5. https://doi.org/10.1016/0002-9394(89)90859-3.
22. Price FW Jr, Whitson WE, Ahad KA, Tavakkoli H. Suprachoroidal hemorrhage in penetrating keratoplasty. Ophthalmic Surg. 1994;25(8):521–5.
23. Ariano ML, Ball SF. Delayed nonexpulsive suprachoroidal hemorrhage after trabeculectomy. Ophthalmic Surg. 1987;18(9):661–6.
24. Becquet F, Caputo G, Mashhour B, Chauvaud D, Pouliquen Y. Management of delayed massive suprachoroidal hemorrhage: a clinical retrospective study. Eur J Ophthalmol. 1996;6(4):393–7.
25. Duncker GI, Rochels R. Delayed suprachoroidal hemorrhage after penetrating keratoplasty. Int Ophthalmol. 1995;19(3):173–6. https://doi.org/10.1007/BF00133734.
26. Ghorayeb G, Khan A, Godley BF. Delayed suprachoroidal hemorrhage after cataract surgery. Retin Cases Brief Rep. 2012;6(4):390–2. https://doi.org/10.1097/ICB.0b013e3182437da2.
27. Jin W, Xing Y, Xu Y, Wang W, Yang A. Management of delayed suprachoriodal haemorrhage after intraocular surgery and trauma. Graefes Arch Clin Exp Ophthalmol. 2014;252(8):1189–93. https://doi.org/10.1007/s00417-013-2550-x.
28. Song W, Zhang Y, Chen H, Du C. Delayed suprachoroidal hemorrhage after cataract surgery: a case report and brief review of literature. Medicine (Baltimore). 2018;97(2):e8697. https://doi.org/10.1097/MD.0000000000008697.
29. Syam PP, Hussain B, Anand N. Delayed suprachoroidal hemorrhage after needle revision of trabeculectomy bleb in a patient with hairy cell leukemia. Am J Ophthalmol. 2003;136(6):1155–7. https://doi.org/10.1016/s0002-9394(03)00574-9.
30. Howe LJ, Bloom P. Delayed suprachoroidal haemorrhage following trabeculectomy bleb needling. Br J Ophthalmol. 1999;83(6):757. https://doi.org/10.1136/bjo.83.6.753f.
31. Aras C, Ozdamar A, Karacorlu M. Suprachoroidal hemorrhage during silicone oil removal in Marfan syndrome. Ophthalmic Surg Lasers. 2000;31(4):337–9.
32. Chandra A, Jazayeri F, Williamson TH. Warfarin in vitreoretinal surgery: a case controlled series. Br J Ophthalmol. 2011;95(7):976–8. https://doi.org/10.1136/bjo.2010.187526.
33. Chandra A, Xing W, Kadhim MR, Williamson TH. Suprachoroidal hemorrhage in pars plana vitrectomy: risk factors and outcomes over 10 years. Ophthalmology. 2014;121(1):311–7. https://doi.org/10.1016/j.ophtha.2013.06.021.
34. Ghoraba HH, Zayed AI. Suprachoroidal hemorrhage as a complication of vitrectomy. Ophthalmic Surg Lasers. 2001;32(4):281–8.
35. Lakhanpal V, Schocket SS, Elman MJ, Dogra MR. Intraoperative massive suprachoroidal hemorrhage during pars plana vitrectomy. Ophthalmology. 1990;97(9):1114–9.
36. Stein JD, Zacks DN, Grossman D, Grabe H, Johnson MW, Sloan FA. Adverse events after pars plana vitrectomy among medicare beneficiaries. Arch Ophthalmol. 2009;127(12):1656–63. https://doi.org/10.1001/archophthalmol.2009.300.
37. Tabandeh H, Flynn HW Jr. Suprachoroidal hemorrhage during pars plana vitrectomy. Curr Opin Ophthalmol. 2001;12(3):179–85.
38. Tabandeh H, Sullivan PM, Smahliuk P, Flynn HW Jr, Schiffman J. Suprachoroidal hemorrhage during pars plana vitrectomy. Risk factors and outcomes. Ophthalmology. 1999;106(2):236–42.
39. Chak M, Williamson TH. Spontaneous suprachoroidal haemorrhage associated with high myopia and aspirin. Eye (Lond). 2003;17(4):525–7. https://doi.org/10.1038/sj.eye.6700388.
40. Masri I, Smith JM, Wride NK, Ghosh S. A rare case of acute angle closure due to spontaneous suprachoroidal haemorrhage secondary to loss of anti-coagulation control: a case report. BMC Ophthalmol. 2018;18(Suppl 1):224. https://doi.org/10.1186/s12886-018-0857-4.
41. Chandra A, Barsam A, Hugkulstone C. A spontaneous suprachoroidal haemorrhage: a case report. Cases J. 2009;2:185. https://doi.org/10.1186/1757-1626-2-185.
42. Cheung AY, David JA, Ober MD. Spontaneous bilateral hemorrhagic choroidal detachments associated with malignant hypertension. Retin Cases Brief Rep. 2017;11(2):175–9. https://doi.org/10.1097/ICB.0000000000000322.

43. Benzimra JD, Johnston RL, Jaycock P, Galloway PH, Lambert G, Chung AK, et al. The cataract national dataset electronic multicentre audit of 55,567 operations: antiplatelet and anticoagulant medications. Eye (Lond). 2009;23(1):10–6. https://doi.org/10.1038/sj.eye.6703069.

44. Williamson TH. Vitreoretinal surgery. 2nd ed. Berlin: Springer; 2013.

45. Jansen MCWH, Haenen JH, van Asten WN, Thien T. Deep Venous thrombosis: a prospective 3-month follow-up using duplex scanning and strain gauge plethysmography. Clin Sci (Lon). 1998;94:651–66.

46. Lakhanpal V. Experimental and clinical observations on massive suprachoroidal hemorrhage. Trans Am Ophthalmol Soc. 1993;91:545–652.

47. Pakravan M, Yazdani S, Afroozifar M, Kouhestani N, Ghassami M, Shahshahan M. An alternative approach for management of delayed suprachoroidal hemorrhage after glaucoma procedures. J Glaucoma. 2014;23(1):37–40. https://doi.org/10.1097/IJG.0b013e31825afb25.

48. Lakhanpal V, Schocket SS, Elman MJ, Nirankari VS. A new modified vitreoretinal surgical approach in the management of massive suprachoroidal hemorrhage. Ophthalmology. 1989;96(6):793–800. https://doi.org/10.1016/s0161-6420(89)32819-3.

49. Fei P, Jin HY, Zhang Q, Li X, Zhao PQ. Tissue plasminogen activator-assisted vitrectomy in the early treatment of acute massive suprachoroidal hemorrhage complicating cataract surgery. Int J Ophthalmol. 2018;11(1):170–1. https://doi.org/10.18240/ijo.2018.01.27.

50. Rezende FA, Kickinger MC, Li G, Prado RF, Regis LG. Transconjunctival drainage of serous and hemorrhagic choroidal detachment. Retina. 2012;32(2):242–9. https://doi.org/10.1097/IAE.0b013e31821c4087.

Choroidal Detachment

Neruban Kumaran and D. Alistair H. Laidlaw

Introduction

Choroidal detachment can be defined as the collection of fluid or blood in the supra-choroidal space, a potential space between choroid and the sclera. Various terms have been used in the literature to describe non-haemorrhagic detachments including choroidal effusion, uveal effusion, ciliochoroidal detachment and ciliochoroidal effusion, which all refer to the same pathology described herein. The suprachoroidal space can be readily identified in nearly half of healthy individuals using enhanced-depth imaging optical coherence tomography (EDI-OCT) and has been suggested to have a mean subfoveal thickness of 36.4 μm [1].

Pathophysiology

As suggested choroidal detachment can either be serous or haemorrhagic in nature.

The leakage of serum from the choroidal vasculature into the suprachoroidal space, resulting in a serous choroidal detachment, can be understood by considering the Starling principle for fluid exchange. The Starling equation is defined as:

N. Kumaran (✉)
St Thomas' Hospital, Guy's and St Thomas' NHS Foundation Trust, London, UK
e-mail: n.kumaran@nhs.net

D. A. H. Laidlaw
St Thomas' Hospital, Guy's and St Thomas' NHS Foundation Trust, London, UK

Maidstone Hospital, Maidstone and Tunbridge Wells NHS Trust, Maidstone, UK

King's College Medical School, London, UK

© The Author(s), under exclusive license to Springer Nature Switzerland AG 2021
S. Saidkasimova, T. H. Williamson (eds.), *Suprachoroidal Space Interventions*,
https://doi.org/10.1007/978-3-030-76853-9_4

$$\text{Net driving pressure} = K_f \left(P_c - P_i \right) - \acute{O} \left(\Pi_c - \Pi_i \right)$$

Where:

K_f = Filtration co-efficient

P_c = capillary hydrostatic pressure

P_i = interstitial hydrostatic pressure

$\acute{O}$ = Staverman's reflection coefficient (correction factor)

Π_c = capillary oncotic pressure

Π_I = interstitial hydrostatic pressure

When considering this equation, the permeability of the choroidal capillaries and the intraocular pressure are reflected in the K_f and P_i, respectively. As such, in the presence of hypotony, the P_i considerably drops, resulting in a flow of fluid out of the capillaries into the suprachoroidal space. Similarly, in an inflammatory state, the capillaries become more leaky with an associated decrease in K_f, again resulting in the flow of fluid from the capillaries into the suprachoroidal space.

In contrast, haemorrhagic choroidal detachment occurs because of a collection of blood, owing to the rupture of long or short posterior ciliary arteries (Fig. 1). They are commonly referred to as suprachoroidal haemorrhage (SCH) and classified on the basis of the size and extent of haemorrhage, relationship to intraocular surgery and/or precipitating events [2]. When described with regards to size, SCH can be described as limited or extensive with the latter often being associated with direct apposition of the inner retinal surfaces, commonly defined as a 'kissing' SCH. Similarly, SCH can be described in relation to surgery. On occasion per operative SCH in eyes with an open wound can be so extensive that there is an expulsion of ocular contents through the surgical wound, categorised as an expulsive choroidal haemorrhage, thereby stressing the importance of closing the wound rapidly in

Fig. 1 Suprachoroidal Haemorrhage. Temporal suprachoroidal haemorrhage and associated subretinal haemorrhage. Image courtesy of Retina Rocks, www.retinarocks.org

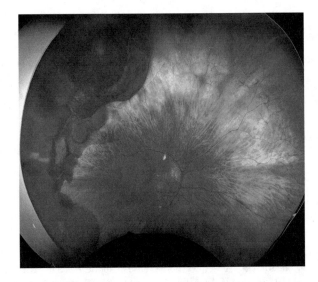

cases where a SCH is suspected. Postoperative or delayed SCH is not typically associated with the expulsion of intraocular contents. However, they may be extensive enough to result in a kissing configuration. Finally, SCHs can also be classified by precipitating events, specifically in the setting of either penetrating or blunt trauma. As might be expected, the greater extent of suprachoroidal haemorrhage and the presence of expulsion are both associated with a poorer visual outcome (see Chap. 3).

Clinical Findings

Serous choroidal detachments may involve some or all of the following features [3]:

1. Choroidal effusion and detachment,
2. Anterior rotation of the ciliary body, with a consequent anterior shift of the lens, a myopic refractive shift and possible secondary angle closure; and ultimately
3. Serous retinal detachment with shifting subretinal fluid.

Typically, serous choroidal detachments may consist of up to four smooth lobes which are limited by the vortex veins as these are firmly anchored to both the choroid and sclera. Furthermore, they are dark in colour (due to the underlying uvea) and have normal overlying retinal vasculature (Fig. 2). A serous choroidal detachment will transilluminate and appear non-echogenic on ultrasound (the opposite being found in suprachoroidal haemorrhage). In cases of retinal apposition, it is impossible to view the posterior pole. Hypotonous maculopathy may also be present.

The secondary angle closure is thought to be caused by associated supraciliary effusions, which either extend anteriorly from the suprachoroidal space or result

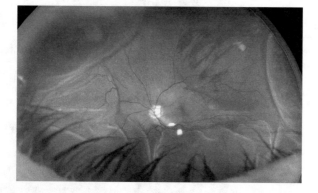

Fig. 2 Serous choroidal detachment secondary to ocular hypotony, following glaucoma filtration surgery. The choroidal detachments are demonstrated as dark in colour with normal overlying retinal vasculature. Subretinal blood is noted as a consequence of a scleral suture during surgery. Image courtesy of Retina Rocks, www.retinarocks.org

from associated ciliary body inflammation [4]. The supraciliary fluid results in detachment and anterior rotation of the ciliary body. Furthermore, the anterior displacement of the choroid, vitreous and subsequently the lens-iris diaphragm results in shallowing of the anterior chamber and potentially appositional angle closure. These features may be imaged using ultrasound biomicroscopy [5]. Such anterior displacement can contribute to intermittent pupil block, but as this is not the primary mechanism of angle closure, iris bombe is often absent.

Consequently, if chronic, the retinal pigment epithelium pump mechanism may fail, resulting in a serous retinal detachment, which in turn is known to increase in volume and viscosity over time.

In comparison to serous choroidal detachments, typically painless, SCH often has an abrupt onset, with considerable pain, headache, nausea and/or vomiting, and decreased visual acuity [2].

In current practice, multi-modal imaging can further help with diagnosis, monitoring and management. B-scan ultrasonography has provided the mainstay of investigations for choroidal detachments (Fig. 3). Firstly, it can be used to differentiate between serous and haemorrhagic choroidal detachments with the latter being more echo dense. Secondly, it allows measurement and documentation of the height of the choroidal detachment. Thirdly, ultrasonography can be used to investigate the dynamics of blood in haemorrhagic choroidal detachments, blood clots within the choroidal detachment initially appear hyper-reflective and with liquefaction over time become less reflective with a swirling echo demonstrating liquefaction. Furthermore, it can also be used to differentiate a choroidal detachment from a rhegmatogenous retinal detachment.

Additionally, widefield fundus photography can be particularly useful in documentation of peripheral choroidal detachment. Both spectral domain and,

Fig. 3 Ultrasound Scan of Serous Choroidal Detachment. Shown is an ultrasound scan of serous choroidal detachment (white arrowheads) in a patient with ocular hypotony following glaucoma surgery

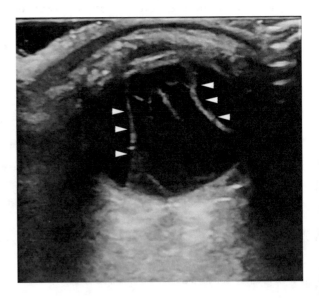

subsequently, swept-source enhanced depth imaging optical coherence tomography (EDI-OCT) suggested great promise with a demonstration of the ability to image the suprachoroidal space. However, to date, the authors are unaware of any studies demonstrating or investigating the utility of EDI-OCT in the diagnosis or management of choroidal detachment.

High-resolution magnetic resonance imaging (MRI) has also been demonstrated to help determine the anatomical location of fluid accumulation, differentiate scleral thickening from choroidal thickening, and identify infiltration and intraocular masses [3].

Differential Diagnoses

Serous choroidal detachment may be confused with exudative retinal detachment, however as suggested above choroidal detachments have a smooth, dark appearance limited by the vortex veins. The retinal pigment epithelium is usually visible through the retina. Serous choroidal detachments are typically immobile and fixed whereas a serous retinal detachment may change distribution with head position (shifting fluid) and will wobble with eye movements. Serous choroidal detachments will transilluminate if a bright point source of light is applied to the sclera, whereas solid choroidal detachments due to haemorrhage or tumour will not.

SCHs need to be differentiated from ocular malignancies/metastases such as choroidal melanoma, ring melanoma, choroiditis and posterior scleritis, all of which can cause a solid choroidal swelling with no choroidal effusion [6].

Causes

The aetiology of serous choroidal detachment can be classified as either inflammatory, hydrostatic or idiopathic (uveal effusion syndrome) in nature (Fig. 4) [6, 7].

Inflammatory Causes of Serous Choroidal Detachment

Inflammatory disorders such as posterior scleritis [8], sympathetic ophthalmia and Vogt-Koyanagi-Harada syndrome [9] are well known to cause serous choroidal detachments. Similarly, serous choroidal detachments have been demonstrated as a presenting feature in an HIV positive patient [10].

Several drugs have been identified as a cause of serous choroidal detachment, including Sulfa agents (Acetazolamide [11], Methazolamide [12], Sulfamethazole [13] and Topiramate [14]), antidepressants (Venlafaxine [15]), chemotherapeutic agents [16] (Gemcitabine and Docetaxel), Losartan [17], Timethoprim, Indapamide

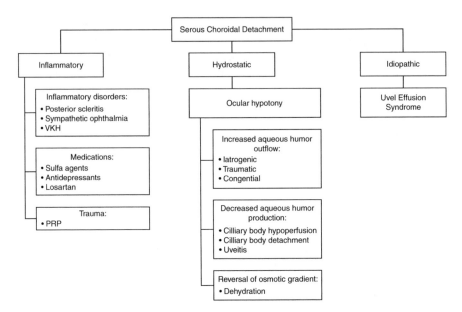

Fig. 4 Causes of serous choroidal detachment. Flow chart demonstrating mechanisms of serous choroidal detachment and selected examples (VKH; Vogt-Koyanagi-Harada disease, PRP; panretinal photocoagulation)

[18], and Bupropion [19]. The aetiology is thought to be a drug-induced ciliary inflammation, which ultimately causes choroidal and ciliary effusions.

Panretinal photocoagulation (PRP) is a recognised cause of serous choroidal detachment. The laser photocoagulation causes disruption of the choriocapilaris, leading to exudation of fluid into the suprachoroidal space, with a transient resolution often seen over the subsequent week [20]. The intensity of the laser burn, dictated by the laser parameters and retinochoroidal absorption is accepted to be the major risk factor for development of such serous detachments following PRP [20]. As such serous choroidal detachment are now much less frequently seen with the popular use of multi-spot lasers with their short duration and smaller diameter burns [21].

Hydrostatic Causes of Serous Choroidal Detachment

The commonest hydrostatic cause for a serous choroidal detachment is ocular hypotony. The causes of ocular hypotony can either be due to increased aqueous humour outflow, decreased aqueous humour production or a reversal of osmotic gradient. Causes for increased aqueous humour outflow include iatrogenic, (surgeries with the potential for an aqueous leak; glaucoma filtering surgeries, phacoemulsification, vitreoretinal surgery) trauma (open globe injury or more commonly a cyclodialysis cleft) or congenital scleral weakness (coloboma). Causes for decreased aqueous humour production include ciliary body hypoperfusion (ocular ischaemic syndrome), ciliary body detachment (proliferative vitreoretinopathy (PVR)), uveitis, aqueous suppressing medications, or cyclodestructive procedures. Other hydrostatic causes for serous choroidal detachment include choroidal or scleral infiltration from systemic conditions such as lymphoma [22] and amyloidosis [23].

Finally, systemic conditions such as severe dehydration [24] can cause a reversal of the osmotic gradient and ocular hypotony.

Uveal Effusion Syndrome (UES)

The diagnosis of Idiopathic uveal effusion or uveal effusion syndrome (UES) is aided by the exclusion of the above causes of choroidal detachment. UES can be further subdivided into those associated with hypermetropia or nanophthalmos and idiopathic [6]. Patients present with a relapsing-remitting course and visual loss. There is an unexplained male preponderance in idiopathic UES.

Nanophthalmos is characterised by its bilateral nature, high hypermetropic refractive error, a normal corneal diameter, a normal crystalline lens, but a short axial length. While there is no agreement on a definitive axial length, less than 21 mm is used by many as a threshold for nanophthalmos [25]. As a result of the normal thickness crystalline lens and short axial length, there is often an anterior displacement of the iris diaphragm, shallow anterior chamber (AC) and chronic angle closure glaucoma. Furthermore, vascular congestion from increased resistance to venous drainage from the eye results in dilated episcleral blood vessels, with blood in Schlemm's canal (which can be visible on gonioscopy). In contrast, the anterior segment in idiopathic UES is often unremarkable.

Posterior segment examination reveals choroidal elevation, chronic macular subretinal fluid and secondary retinal pigment epithelium (RPE) changes which are described as a leopard spot fundus. Subretinal fluid in such cases is found to have high concentrations of serum proteins and in particular, albumin [26, 27]. In common with other causes of serous retinal detachment, it has a smooth convex surface and will demonstrate shifting fluid due to its gravity dependent nature.

Different mechanisms have been proposed with regards to the pathogenesis of UES.

1. Thickening of the sclera resulting in relative obstruction to venous outflow via the vortex veins, in turn causing congestion of the choriocapillaris and subsequent uveal effusion [28].
2. Reduced transscleral diffusion of protein causing impairment of normal egress of protein across the sclera, and subsequent retention of osmotically active protein and thence fluid in the suprachoroidal space [26, 29].
3. Chronic hypotony causing uveal effusion in non-nanophthalmic eyes [30].
4. Increased choroidal vessel permeability [31].

With both clinical and experimental data supporting each hypothesis there is an acceptance that all of the above can contribute to the pathogenesis of UES with a variation in the relative contribution of each in any individual [6].

Multiple histological studies have been undertaken on sclera in the context of nanophthalmia. They have demonstrated a thickened sclera, an interwoven, irregular arrangement of collagen bundles, with abnormal deposition of proteoglycan GAG between collagen bundles [32, 33]. Furthermore, it has been proposed that UES represents a form of ocular mucopolysaccharidosis with an abnormal accumulation of dermatan sulphate and chondroitin sulphate [34].

On the basis of the above, it has been proposed that UES can be further divided into three types [35]:

- Type 1: Nanophthalmic eyes with a small eyeball (average axial length 16 mm) and high hypermetropia (average + 16 diopters).
- Type 2: Non-nanophthalmic eyes with clinically abnormal sclera; normal eyeball size (average axial length 21 mm) and a small refractive error.
- Type 3: Non-nanophthalmic eyes with the clinically normal sclera and a normal eyeball size.

This group further suggest that types 1 and 2 respond better to surgical interventions similar to the 'scleral decompression window' described below.

Management

Management of choroidal detachment is targeted towards the underlying cause.

In SCH, specific clinical features influence the decision to consider surgical drainage (see below) such as the presence of retinal detachment, central retinal apposition, vitreous incarceration into a wound, breakthrough vitreous haemorrhage, raised intraocular pressure (IOP), retained lens material from cataract surgery, and intractable eye pain [2]. Central retinal apposition was historically considered an absolute indication for surgery as it was thought that it would result in an irreversibly closed funnel configuration retinal detachment due to the retina sticking to itself on its apposed inner surfaces [36]. However, more recent studies have demonstrated this not to be the case [37]. The management of suprachoroidal haemorrhage is discussed in greater detail in Chap. 3.

Inflammatory causes for serous choroidal detachments can be managed by targeting the underlying condition, often with the use of systemic immunosuppression. Drug-induced serous choroidal detachments gradually resolve on cessation of the causative medication, in consultation with the appropriate physician.

Similarly, hydrostatic causes for serous choroidal detachments can be managed by addressing the underlying cause. The risk of ocular hypotony arising from glaucoma surgery can be mitigated peri-operatively. When undertaking trabeculectomy, this can be achieved with measures that prevent over-drainage either into the subconjunctival space (by sufficiently suturing the scleral flap) or an external leakage through a conjunctival defect onto the ocular surface. The latter is managed with careful conjunctival suturing and careful use of antimetabolites for adequate conjunctival limbal healing. The tube can be ligated, or a two-stage surgery performed to allow a fibrous capsule to form around the plate when non-valved glaucoma drainage devices are employed in order to avoid early postoperative hypotony [38].

Furthermore, in unique situations considered to be at high-risk of choroidal detachment, such as nanophthalmos, prophylactic sclerotomies can be performed. Whilst now rarely performed such prophylactic sclerotomies can be used as a routine part of cataract surgery in nanophthalmic eyes [39].

The following technique has been described by multiple groups for drainage in the context of postoperative SCH or ocular hypotony associated serous choroidal detachment [40, 41]. Preoperatively the location of maximal choroidal detachment should be identified. The AC is reformed either with balanced salt solution using an AC maintainer or with viscoelastic. Continuous infusion is imperative to encourage drainage and to avoid worse hypotony and SCH. A tangential conjunctival incision is made 3–6 mm from the limbus in the desired quadrant, with cautery for haemostasis. A 2–3 mm radial sclerotomy is made 3–4 mm from the limbus. Spontaneous drainage should occur, however further flow can be encouraged by opening the lips of the incision. The fluid may be clear and yellowish in serous choroidal detachment or dark red with blood clots in SCH. The sclerotomy site can be left open, and the conjunctival wound closed. This can be repeated in another quadrant if necessary and/or performed with concomitant operations such as bleb revision or cataract surgery. The drainage aspect of this method has more recently been modified with groups demonstrating success with the use of 20 gauge and 25 gauge trocars inserted transconjunctivally, 7 mm from the limbus [42] and also via the pars plana [43]. These have the additional benefit of conjunctival preservation, especially useful in eyes with concomitant conjunctival thinning/scarring from previous antimetabolite usage during glaucoma surgery.

Where surgical interventions have caused an increased aqueous outflow, these can be either monitored for spontaneous resolution or the source of the leak surgically closed. One should, however, be aware of the risk of secondary SCH.

The management of cyclodialysis clefts is often tailored according to the size of the cleft. Smaller clefts (less than two clock hours) can be managed with either high powered laser to the cleft or cryopexy over the cleft, to create swelling and subsequent adhesion. Larger clefts may require transscleral suturing with a non-absorbable suture [44]. One should be aware of rebound secondary glaucoma from the damaged iridocorneal angle.

Decreased aqueous humour production can be caused by tractional ciliary detachment. The commonest instance of this would be in patients with a PVR retinal detachment. A cyclitic membrane is an extreme example of such tractional detachment. Dissection of the cicatricial membrane has been described, however, this is usually unsuccessful and is now rarely performed.

Furthermore, atrophy of the ciliary processes from cyclodestructive procedures, chronic uveitis and damage to the ciliary vessels and nerves with the deeper penetrating diode laser has been described. Management in such scenarios includes the use of cohesive viscoelastic such as Healon GV (Johnson & Johnson Vision, Florida, USA) in the anterior chamber or vitreous cavity, or pars plana vitrectomy with the insertion of silicone oil to maintain ocular volume [45, 46].

As UES is caused by abnormal scleral composition, medical treatment is ineffective. As such 'scleral decompression windows' have been described [6, 26]. A 360-degree conjunctival peritomy is performed. A half to two-thirds scleral thickness rectangular (5 × 7 mm) section of sclera is dissected, centred 1–2 mm anterior to the equator with the long axis oriented circumferentially, taking care to avoid the areas anterior to the vortex veins. A linear 2 mm sclerostomy is then made in the centre of each sclerectomy site, without choroidal perforation. These windows can be performed in two to four quadrants as appropriate. In a study by Jackson et al. investigating this approach in UES, 7 out of 14 subjects demonstrated complete resolution of choroidal effusion with one operation, three partial resolution and failure in 4 subjects [29].

References

1. Yiu G, Pecen P, Sarin N, Chiu SJ, Farsiu S, Mruthyunjaya P, et al. Characterisation of the choroid-scleral junction and suprachoroidal layer in healthy individuals on enhanced-depth imaging optical coherence tomography. JAMA Ophthalmol. 2014;132(2):174–81.
2. Chu TG, Green RL. Suprachoroidal hemorrhage. Surv Ophthalmol. 1999;43(6):471–86.
3. Shah PR, Yohendran J, Hunyor AP, Grigg JR, McCluskey PJ. Uveal effusion: clinical features, management, and visual outcomes in a retrospective case series. J Glaucoma. 2016;25(4):e329–35.
4. Yang JG, Li JJ, Tian H, Li YH, Gong YJ, Su AL, et al. Uveal effusion following acute primary angle-closure: a retrospective case series. Int J Ophthalmol. 2017;10(3):406–12.
5. Kishi A, Nao-i N, Sawada A. Ultrasound biomicroscopic findings of acute angle-closure glaucoma in Vogt-Koyanagi-Harada syndrome. Am J Ophthalmol. 1996;122(5):735–7.
6. Elagouz M, Stanescu-Segall D, Jackson TL. Uveal effusion syndrome. Surv Ophthalmol. 2010;55(2):134–45.
7. Diep MQ, Madigan MC. Choroidal detachments: what do optometrists need to know? Clin Exp Optom. 2019;102(2):116–25.
8. McCluskey PJ, Watson PG, Lightman S, Haybittle J, Restori M, Branley M. Posterior scleritis: clinical features, systemic associations, and outcome in a large series of patients. Ophthalmology. 1999;106(12):2380–6.
9. Yang P, Liu X, Zhou H, Guo W, Zhou C, Kijlstra A. Vogt-Koyanagi-Harada disease presenting as acute angle closure glaucoma at onset. Clin Exp Ophthalmol. 2011;39(7):639–47.
10. Nash RW, Lindquist TD. Bilateral angle-closure glaucoma associated with uveal effusion: presenting sign of HIV infection. Surv Ophthalmol. 1992;36(4):255–8.
11. Man X, Costa R, Ayres BM, Moroi SE. Acetazolamide-induced bilateral ciliochoroidal effusion syndrome in plateau Iris configuration. Am J Ophthalmol Case Rep. 2016;3:14–7.
12. Kwon SJ, Park DH, Shin JP. Bilateral transient myopia, angle-closure glaucoma, and choroidal detachment induced by methazolamide. Jpn J Ophthalmol. 2012;56(5):515–7.
13. Postel EA, Assalian A, Epstein DL. Drug-induced transient myopia and angle-closure glaucoma associated with supraciliary choroidal effusion. Am J Ophthalmol. 1996;122(1):110–2.
14. Craig JE, Ong TJ, Louis DL, Wells JM. Mechanism of topiramate-induced acute-onset myopia and angle closure glaucoma. Am J Ophthalmol. 2004;137(1):193–5.

15. de Guzman MH, Thiagalingam S, Ong PY, Goldberg I. Bilateral acute angle closure caused by supraciliary effusions associated with venlafaxine intake. Med J Aust. 2005;182(3):121–3.
16. Kord Valeshabad A, Mieler WF, Setlur V, Thomas M, Shahidi M. Posterior segment toxicity after gemcitabine and docetaxel chemotherapy. Optometry Vis Sci. 2015;92(5):e110–3.
17. Lipa RK, Sánchez ME, Ordovas CA, Aragües AR, Borque CG. Circumscribed ciliochoroidal effusion presenting as an acute angle closure attack. J Ophthalmic Vis Res. 2017;12(1):117–9.
18. Végh M, Hári-Kovács A, Réz K, Tapasztó B, Szabó A, Facskó A. Indapamide-induced transient myopia with supraciliary effusion: case report. BMC Ophthalmol. 2013;13:58.
19. Takusagawa HL, Hunter RS, Jue A, Pasquale LR, Chen TC. Bilateral uveal effusion and angle-closure glaucoma associated with bupropion use. Arch Ophthalmol. 2012;130(1):120–2.
20. Yuki T, Kimura Y, Nanbu S, Kishi S, Shimizu K. Ciliary body and choroidal detachment after laser photocoagulation for diabetic retinopathy. A high-frequency ultrasound study. Ophthalmology. 1997;104(8):1259–64.
21. Natesh S, Ranganath A, Harsha K, Yadav NK, Bhujang BS. Choroidal detachment after PASCAL photocoagulation. Can J Ophthalmol J Can d'ophtalmologie. 2011;46(1):91.
22. Holz FG, Boehmer HV, Mechtersheimer G, Ott G, Völcker HE. Uveal non-Hodgkin's lymphoma with epibulbar extension simulating choroidal effusion syndrome. Retina (Philadelphia, Pa). 1999;19(4):343–6.
23. Liew SC, McCluskey PJ, Parker G, Taylor RF. Bilateral uveal effusion associated with scleral thickening due to amyloidosis. Arch Ophthalmol. 2000;118(9):1293–5.
24. Murthy G, Kamat SA. Ocular hypotony following acute gastroenteritis. J Assoc Physicians India. 1982;30(2):119.
25. Carricondo PC, Andrade T, Prasov L, Ayres BM, Moroi SE. Nanophthalmos: a review of the clinical spectrum and genetics. J Ophthalmol. 2018;2018:2735465.
26. Gass JD. Uveal effusion syndrome. A new hypothesis concerning pathogenesis and technique of surgical treatment. Retina (Philadelphia, Pa). 1983;3(3):159–63.
27. Brockhurst RJ, Lam KW. Uveal effusion. II. Report of a case with analysis of subretinal fluid. Arch Ophthalmol. 1973;90(5):399–401.
28. Calhoun FP Jr. The management of glaucoma in nanophthalmos. Trans Am Ophthalmol Soc. 1975;73:97–122.
29. Jackson TL, Hussain A, Morley AM, Sullivan PM, Hodgetts A, El-Osta A, et al. Scleral hydraulic conductivity and macromolecular diffusion in patients with uveal effusion syndrome. Invest Ophthalmol Vis Sci. 2008;49(11):5033–40.
30. Daniele S, Schepens CL. Can chronic bulbar hypotony be responsible for uveal effusion? Report of two cases. Ophthalmic Surg. 1989;20(12):872–5.
31. Kumar A, Kedar S, Singh RP. The indocyanine green findings in idiopathic uveal effusion syndrome. Indian J Ophthalmol. 2002;50(3):217–9.
32. Trelstad RL, Silbermann NN, Brockhurst RJ. Nanophthalmic sclera. Ultrastructural, histochemical, and biochemical observations. Arch Ophthalmol. 1982;100(12):1935–8.
33. Yue BY, Duvall J, Goldberg MF, Puck A, Tso MO, Sugar J. Nanophthalmic sclera. Morphologic and tissue culture studies. Ophthalmology. 1986;93(4):534–41.
34. Forrester JV, Lee WR, Kerr PR, Dua HS. The uveal effusion syndrome and trans-scleral flow. Eye (London, England). 1990;4(Pt 2):354–65.
35. Uyama M, Takahashi K, Kozaki J, Tagami N, Takada Y, Ohkuma H, et al. Uveal effusion syndrome: clinical features, surgical treatment, histologic examination of the sclera, and pathophysiology. Ophthalmology. 2000;107(3):441–9.
36. Berrocal JA. Adhesion of the retina secondary to large choroidal detachment as a cause of failure in retinal detachment surgery. Mod Probl Ophthalmol. 1979;20:51–2.
37. Chu TG, Cano MR, Green RL, Liggett PE, Lean JS. Massive suprachoroidal hemorrhage with central retinal apposition. A clinical and echographic study. Arch Ophthalmol. 1991;109(11):1575–81.
38. Reddy A, Salim S. Choroidal effusions EyeNet Magazine: American Academy of Ophthalmology; 2012. https://www.aao.org/eyenet/article/choroidal-effusions.

39. Rajendrababu S, Babu N, Sinha S, Balakrishnan V, Vardhan A, Puthuran GV, et al. A randomized controlled trial comparing outcomes of cataract surgery in nanophthalmos with and without prophylactic Sclerostomy. Am J Ophthalmol. 2017;183:125–33.
40. Bellows AR, Chylack LT Jr, Hutchinson BT. Choroidal detachment. Clinical manifestation, therapy and mechanism of formation. Ophthalmology. 1981;88(11):1107–15.
41. WuDunn D, Ryser D, Cantor LB. Surgical drainage of choroidal effusions following glaucoma surgery. J Glaucoma. 2005;14(2):103–8.
42. Rezende FA, Kickinger MC, Li G, Prado RF, Regis LG. Transconjunctival drainage of serous and hemorrhagic choroidal detachment. Retina (Philadelphia, Pa). 2012;32(2):242–9.
43. Safuri S, Bar-David L, Barak Y. Minimally invasive technique for choroidal fluid drainage. Clin Ophthalmol (Auckland, NZ). 2020;14:1955–8.
44. Ioannidis AS, Bunce C, Barton K. The evaluation and surgical management of cyclodialysis clefts that have failed to respond to conservative management. Br J Ophthalmol. 2014;98(4):544–9.
45. Küçükerdönmez C, Beutel J, Bartz-Schmidt KU, Gelisken F. Treatment of chronic ocular hypotony with intraocular application of sodium hyaluronate. Br J Ophthalmol. 2009;93(2):235–9.
46. Kapur R, Birnbaum AD, Goldstein DA, Tessler HH, Shapiro MJ, Ulanski LJ, et al. Treating uveitis-associated hypotony with pars plana vitrectomy and silicone oil injection. Retina (Philadelphia, Pa). 2010;30(1):140–5.

Suprachoroidal Space and Glaucoma

Leon Au and Antonio Fea

Introduction

Glaucoma is a condition of optic neuropathy leading to progressive visual field loss often associated with raised intraocular pressure (IOP). The aqueous humour is formed by the ciliary processes as a result of active transport of solutes by the double layered ciliary epithelium. After entering the anterior chamber, it is mostly drains away via the trabecular meshwork (TM) into the Schlemm's canal, then passes via the collector channels into the episcleral veins. This constitutes the conventional or trabecular outflow. However, a second drainage pathway exists where aqueous humour passes from the anterior chamber through the ciliary muscle into the supraciliary and suprachoroidal space [1]. This occurs as there is no epithelial barrier between the anterior chamber and the ciliary muscle. Fluid in the suprachoroidal space is thought to exit the globe either via diffusion through the sclera or drainage via the choroidal capillaries into the vortex veins, or both. This is often referred to as the unconventional or uveoscleral outflow. [1, 2]

The treatment of glaucoma continues to focus on lowering the intraocular pressure by manipulation of the aqueous inflow and outflow mechanism. Traditional glaucoma medications such as beta-blockers and carbonic anhydrase inhibitors aim to lower IOP by reduction of aqueous production. More permanent cyclo-destruction is achieved surgically using cryotherapy and diode laser. Selective laser trabeculoplasty aims to increase conventional outflow by increasing aqueous transfer through

L. Au (✉)
Manchester Royal Eye Hospital, Manchester, UK
e-mail: Leon.Au@mft.nhs.uk

A. Fea
University of Turin, Turin, Italy

S. Saidkasimova, T. H. Williamson (eds.), *Suprachoroidal Space Interventions*,
https://doi.org/10.1007/978-3-030-76853-9_5

the TM, while TM bypassing surgical micro-devices can be inserted at the angle to achieve similar result. Of course, classic glaucoma filtration surgery like trabeculectomy or glaucoma drainage implant lowers IOP dramatically by diverting aqueous into the subconjunctival space. The uveoscleral outflow pathway has also been the subject of great interest in the quest for the ideal glaucoma treatment. Both pharmacological and surgical approach to increase uveoscleral pathway has been explored over the years and met with variable success.

Pharmacological Manipulation of the Uveoscleral Outflow

The principal site of uveoscleral outflow resistance intraocularly is the ciliary muscle [2]. Cholinergic agents, like pilocarpine, cause contraction of the ciliary muscle making it less permeable to aqueous and reduce the uveoscleral outflow. Paradoxically, since the ciliary muscle fibres are attached to the trabecular meshwork, ciliary contraction leads to the dilation of the Schlemm's canal and an increase in the conventional outflow [2]. Hence pilocarpine was used in the past as glaucoma treatment, but its side effect and the lack of efficacy compared to newer treatment has rendered it useful only in a specific situation like angle closure glaucoma. On the other hand, relaxation of the ciliary muscle, with atropine, has the opposite effect of the widening of spaces between muscle bundle and increasing the uveoscleral outflow. Adrenergic drugs, like epinephrine, also demonstrated an increase in the uveoscleral outflow in monkeys although the exact mechanism was unclear [2].

Prostaglandin Analogues

The introduction of prostaglandin PGF2alpha analogues (e.g. latanoprost, travaprost and bimatoprost) marked a significant advancement in the management of glaucoma. This group of medication offers remarkable IOP reduction [3, 4]. One unique feature of the uveoscleral outflow system is its insensitivity to the pressure difference that drives the flow; it was reported that as IOP increases between 4 mmHg and 35 mmHg the uveoscleral outflow remains almost constant, compared to the increase in the conventional trabecular outflow [3]. However, the introduction of prostaglandin appears to relax the ciliary muscle as well as causing remodelling of the extracellular matrix within the muscle, enlarging spaces between the fibre bundles and thereby reducing its resistance to the outflow and increasing the pressure sensitivity of this outflow system [4]. Since its commercial introduction prostaglandin eyedrops have become the first line glaucoma therapy worldwide.

Surgical Exploration of Suprachoroidal Space in Glaucoma

Cyclodialysis Cleft

Since the largest resistance lies at the ciliary muscle, separation of the ciliary body results in an unimpeded outflow of the aqueous from the anterior chamber into the suprachoroidal space. Significant IOP reduction results from the increased uveoscleral outflow as well as the reduced aqueous production by the detached ciliary body [5]. Cyclodialysis cleft is the most often encountered after trauma or accidental damage during intraocular surgery [6, 7]. Clinically patient would often present with hypotony, sometimes accompanied by shallowing of the anterior chamber. Gonioscopy reveals a particularly recessed angle where ciliary fibre is torn off its attachment, revealing the underlying pearly white sclera and a dark cleft. However, due to the softer globe and shallow anterior chamber, it can be difficult to visualise the cyclodialysis cleft. An intracameral injection of viscoelastic to deepen the anterior chamber can be useful to aid gonioscopy [6, 7]. Modern imaging techniques like ultrasound biomicroscopy (UBM) and anterior segment OCT (AS-OCT) is crucial in confirming the diagnosis. (Fig. 1) AS-OCT has an advantage over UBM in being non-invasive and non-contact while UBM can be difficult in a tender, soft eye. It is also easier to delineate the clock-hours of the cleft with AS-OCT over the handheld UBM.

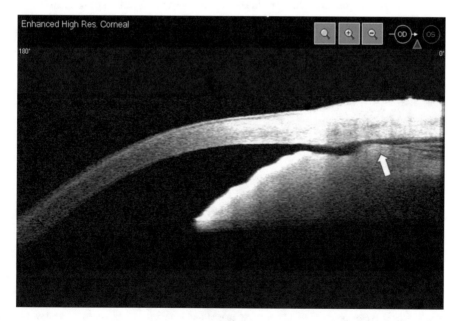

Fig. 1 AS-OCT demonstrating significant cyclodialysis cleft (arrow) and shallowing of anterior chamber

Once the cyclodialysis is identified and its extent is localised, closure can be achieved with medical, laser or surgical treatment depending on the size of the cleft, both in terms of the width, in clock-hours, as well as the height of the ciliary body separation from the sclera. Initial treatment for shallow, less than three clock hours cleft is often topical cycloplegic like atropine 1% for a few weeks [6, 7]. If the cleft does not close, high energy localised diode laser or cryotherapy can be applied to the cleft area to induce inflammation and scaring [6, 7]. For large height cleft of more than four clock-hours, surgical repair is often required. Direct cyclopexy remains the most definitive treatment where under a partial thickness scleral flap the ciliary body is reattached to the sclera by multiple sutures [6, 7]. (Fig. 2) Other ab-interno techniques have been reported including the use of capsule tension ring in the sulcus, large haptic PMMA lens implant orientated towards the cleft and pars plana vitrectomy with internal gas tamponade [8–10].

Cyclodialysis as Surgical Treatment

Cyclodialysis, as a treatment for certain cases of open angle glaucoma and aphakic glaucoma, was first introduced by ophthalmologist Leopold Heine in 1905 [11]. The technique was debated at the time and various modifications were reported [12–14]. Essentially it consists of a full thickness scleral incision or trephination near or behind the rectus muscle insertion to expose the suprachoroidal space [11–14]. A

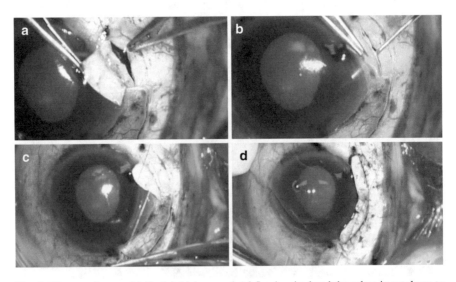

Fig. 2 Direct cyclopexy. (**a**) Partial thickness scleral flap is raised and the sclera is cut down to expose choroid. (**b**) Cleft is identified with a cannula. (**c**) Direct suturing with non-absorbable suture closing the sclera and underlying ciliary body at the same time. (**d**) Multiple interrupted sutures with close spacing to ensure good cleft closure

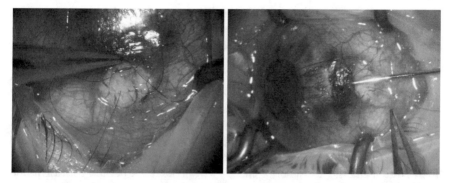

Fig. 3 Cyclodialysis procedure through a scleral incision 3 mm from limbus. A cyclodialysis spatula is passed into anterior chamber to create a cleft. *(Courtesy of Cecilia Fenerty, MD)*

cyclodialysis spatula is introduced carefully into the space and advanced forward until it reaches the anterior chamber. Side way sweeping motion bluntly detach the ciliary body from the sclera over the desired number of clock hours creating a cleft. (Fig. 3) Successful long term IOP control was reported together with unpredictability and complications of haemorrhage, hypotony and failure due to synechia closure of the cleft [13, 14]. Cyclodialysis as a sole surgical treatment for glaucoma is no longer in practice although more modern reports of combining cyclodialysis with trabeculectomy exist in the literature with favourable outcome [15].

Glaucoma Implants for Suprachoroidal Space

Although some success was reported with cyclodialysis as a solo procedure to reduce IOP, failure often occurred as a result of fibrotic closure of the cleft. Hence attempts were made to insert different implants and spacers into the cleft to maintain patency and aid efficacy. Gills described the use of plastic tubing in primate and human and concluded that the reduction of IOP was primarily due to reduced aqueous production rather than increased uveoscleral outflow [16, 17]. Other materials have been reported since including the use of scleral strip, Krupin valve and Ologen implants [15, 18, 19]. Few commercial drainage devices were launched over the last decade focusing on uveoscleral drainage with variable success.

SOLX Gold Microshunt

The SOLX gold microshunt (SOLX inc. Waltham, MA, USA) was one of the first glaucoma drainage devices specifically designed to drain into suprachoroidal space. The device was manufactured with industrial grade 24-karat gold which was thought to be inert with good biocompatibility to the human eye. The gold microshunt (GMS) was 3.2 mm wide, 5.2 mm long and was T-shaped with the slimmer round end designed to sit in the anterior chamber. Later a revised version GMS plus was developed with a longer body of 5.5 mm and slightly increased thickness. The device was composed of two leaflets fused together concealing multiple microchannels within the body to allow egress of aqueous into the suprachoroidal space. The device was implanted ab-externo after a limited conjunctival peritomy. A 95% depth scleral incision was made around 3 mm from the limbus and dissection was performed using a crescent knife both anteriorly up to the scleral spur as well as 2 mm posteriorly into the suprachoroidal space. The device was then inserted with the front portion entering the anterior chamber while the back-portion slided into the suprachoroidal space. The scleral incision is sutured watertight to avoid bleb formation [20]. (Fig. 4).

The first pilot study by Melamed et al. was published in 2009, demonstrating one year follow up outcomes of 38 patients with advanced glaucoma [20]. GMS implantation resulted in a mean of 9 mmHg IOP reduction from 27.6 (SD 4.7) to 18.2 (SD 4.6) mmHg, while 79% of patients achieved IOP >5 and < 22 mm Hg, with the majority achieving that with antiglaucoma medication at the last follow up. Figus

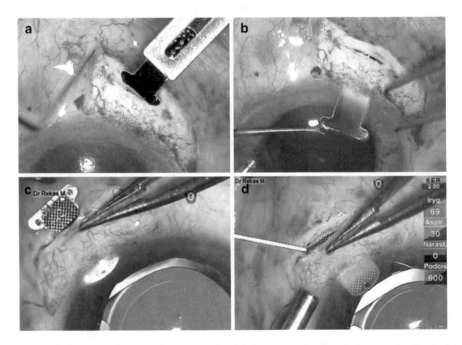

Fig. 4 Implantation of the GMS and GMS plus. (**a**) GMS plus: placement of the proximal part of the implant in the anterior chamber, (**b**) GMS plus: placement of the distal part of the implant in the suprachoroidal space, (**c**) GMS: placement of the proximal part of the implant in the anterior chamber, (**d**) GMS: placement of the distal part of the implant in the suprachoroidal space. (*Courtesy of Merek Rekas, MD*)

et al. reported their two-year outcome in 55 patients with previous failed glaucoma surgery. The qualified success rate (IOP >5 and < 22 mmHg on antiglaucoma medication) at two years was 67.3% with a mean post-operative IOP at 13.7 ± 2.98 mmHg, a statistically significant reduction from the preoperative IOP of 27.6 ± 6.9 mmHg. The medication was also reduced by 1.1 drop [21]. Skaat and colleagues conducted a five year comparative study of the GMS against the Ahmed glaucoma valve which was published in 2016 [22]. In this study patients with refractory glaucoma (previous failed glaucoma surgery) were randomised into having GMS, GMS plus or Ahmed valve implantation. All three arms demonstrated significant IOP reduction and similar success, but the sample size was small and the final mean IOP of the groups were between 17-19 mmHg; a target IOP that would be deemed too high for this group of patients with refractory glaucoma. Efficacy of the GMS was not universally reported. Heuber et al. retrospectively reviewed 31 GMS implanted for refractory glaucoma and showed a very disappointing 97% surgical failure rate, either due to suboptimal IOP (outside 5-22 mmHg), serious complications or requiring additional glaucoma surgery [23]. In fact, 77% of eyes required additional surgery within the first year. Overall complication of GMS included hyphaema, hypotony, corneal decompensation and erosions [24]. Failure of these implants were found to be related to connective tissue proliferation, wrapping around the GMS and obstructing the micro-channels [25] (Fig. 5). Currently the SOLX gold microshunt is no longer available commercially, and the company appears to have ceased trading.

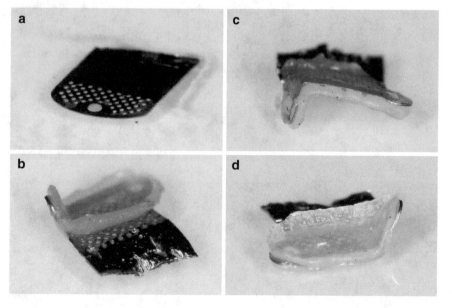

Fig. 5 Failed explanted SOLX gold microshunt demonstrating fibrotic tissue obstructing the device. *(Courtesy of Merek Rekas, MD)*

Cypass Suprachoroidal Microshunt

The Cypass microshunt was developed by Transcend Medical, USA which subsequently was acquired by Alcon, USA and launched globally as the first minimally invasive glaucoma surgical (MIGS) device to target suprachoroidal/supraciliary drainage. The device is cylindrical in shape, made of a nonbiodegradable polyimide material that is demonstrated to have excellent biocompatibility [26]. The semiflexible implants is 6.35 mm long, with a 0.43 mm in outer diameter and a lumen size of 0.30 mm. It has three retention rings at the anterior chamber end and multiple fenestrations along its shaft. The device is designed to sit in the supraciliary space draining aqueous from the anterior chamber into the suprachoroidal space [26] (Fig. 6).

Cypass microshunt is a straight device but comes pre-loaded in an introducer with a slightly curved guidewire to aid insertion (Fig. 7). The device is inserted ab-interno with the aid of intraoperative gonioscopy. After filling the anterior chamber with cohesive viscoelastic the angle is visualised with a gonioprism (e.g. Swan-Jacob lens). The device is introduced through a temporal clear corneal incision, across the anterior chamber towards the nasal angle. It is then gently inserted just

Fig. 6 Cypass microshunt

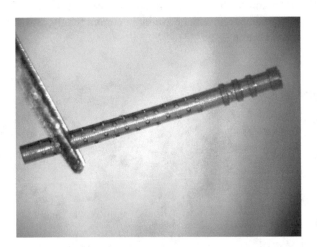

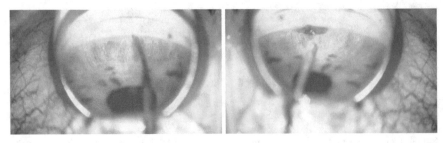

Fig. 7 Cypass insertion via ab-internal approach with 1 retention ring visible at the end of surgery

below the scleral spur, sliding posteriorly into the supraciliary space until the level retention rings. The device is then released from the introducer and gently tapped in until ideally only 1 retention ring is visible.

Hoh et al. reported one of the earlier case series of Cypass microshunt in clinical settings. A total of 82 patients reached a two-year follow up [26]. The group was divided into cohort one, where preop IOP was uncontrolled at over 22 mmHg, and cohort two, where preop IOP was deemed to be controlled. For cohort one, the IOP showed a significant reduction from 25.5 mmHg preop to 16 mmHg after 24 months (p < 0.0001). For the controlled cohort two there was no change in IOP, but the number of glaucoma medication was significantly reduced from 2.0 ± 0.9 to 1.1 ± 1.1 at two years (p < 0.0001). The complication rate was reasonably low, with 15.4% of patients experiencing early post-operative hypotony, while 11% of patients ultimately required further glaucoma surgeries.

The Cypass microshunt received FDA approval in 2016 based on its pivotal COMPASS trial where 505 patients with primary open angle glaucoma (POAG) were treated with Cypass combined with phacoemulsification vs phacoemulsification alone. [27] This was a two-year prospective multicentred randomised controlled trial with 373 patients receiving the Cypass and 131 as control. Success criteria were defined as greater than 20% reduction of washed out IOP. This was achieved in 60% of the control group while adding a Cypass increased that to 77%. The Cypass offered an extra 2 mmHg of IOP reduction after medication washed out. IOP was maintained <21 mmHg with no medication in 85% of the Cypass group patients compared to only 59% in the control group. Medication count was also three times higher in the control arm. Adverse events were low with a small number of hyphaema, transient hypotony, malposition and peripheral anterior synechiae obstructing the device [27].

The Cypass was also evaluated as a standalone procedure in patients with failed topical treatment in the multicentred DUETTE trial. Garcia-Feijoo and colleagues recruited 65 eyes with uncontrolled IOP for filtration surgery with a single Cypass implanted without phacoemulsification. At 12 months mean IOP was reduced from 24.5 ± 2.8 mm Hg to 16.4 ± 5.5 mm Hg, while medication was also reduced from 2.2 to 1.4 drops. More importantly, 83% of eyes were saved from needing a further glaucoma surgery at 12 months. Kerr et al. reported its use in 20 patients with previous failed trabeculectomy or tube surgery, demonstrating a 33.7% reduction in IOP down to 14.9 ± 4.3 mmHg and a 56% reduction in medication [28].

The life of the Cypass, however, was cut short when Alcon announced a global voluntary withdrawal of the device in August 2018 [29]. After evaluating the extended COMPASS trial data at 5 years (termed COMPASS-XT), a significant central endothelial loss was found in the Cypass group compared to the control; at 60 months, significant endothelial cell loss (>30%) was more common in the Cypass group (27.2%) compared with the control group (10%). When evaluating the position of the Cypass stent, it was found that if the device was not pushed in well, the amount of endothelial cell loss increased. Devices with 2 or 3 retention rings visible on gonioscopy had around 10% cell loss at 5 year compared to around 2% in fully implanted devices (Fig. 8).

Fig. 8 Cypass implant, showing 3 exposed retention rings with increased risk of endothelial cell loss, can be trimmed ab-interno using 20G retinal scissors

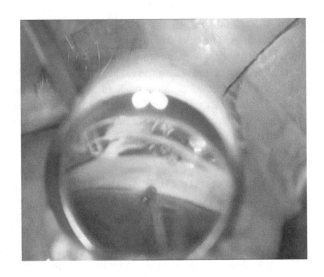

Future Suprachoroidal Glaucoma Devices

There are two other suprachoroidal devices, which are less known: the iStent Supra and the MINIject. Both are implanted ab-interno and may be placed in conjunction with cataract surgery or as a standalone procedure. Both are currently undergoing pre-clinical evaluation and are not yet commercially available.

iStent Supra

The iStent Supra (Glaukos, USA) has been CE marked for use in Europe and is a device very similar in concept to the Cypass microshunt [30]. The iStent Supra (Fig.9) is a 4 mm ridged tube with a lumen diameter that varies between 0.16 mm and 0.17 mm, while the outside diameter varies between 0.3 and 0.4 mm that is curved to conform to the contour of the globe within the suprachoroidal space. The device is made of polyethersulfone, which promises favourable biomaterial interaction with minimal fibrosis, and titanium, with a heparin-coated lumen. Retention ridges along the shaft are present on the surface of the stent to hold it in place. The mode of delivery is almost identical to that of the Cypass described above. The significant differences between Cypass and iStent Supra are material (Polyimide vs Polyethersulfone), the lumen size (300 vs 165 μm), and the length (6.35 vs 4 mm). Furthermore, the iStent Supra is curved and has retention features not limited to the iris root but to its whole part sitting into the suprachoroidal space.

The information on the clinical safety and efficacy of this device is relatively modest and mainly limited to non-peer reviewed presentations. 73 POAG patients with a mean preoperative medicated diurnal IOP of 20.4 mmHg (unmedicated of

Fig. 9 Design of the iStent Supra *(Courtesy of Glaukos, USA)*

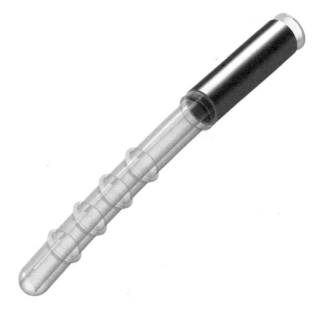

24.8 mmHg) were implanted with the iStent Supra and 42 of them were followed through 12 months; of the latter, 98% met the primary endpoint of a 20% reduction in IOP with one medication (Travoprost). The mean IOP decreased by 47% to 13.2 mmHg. Of equal importance, there were no documented adverse events during the study [31].

The iStent Supra has also been used in combination with other MIGS devices (trabecular micro-bypass stents) in POAG patients refractory to conventional filtration surgery and medication. Out of 80 subjects with persistently elevated IOP following trabeculectomy despite the use of medications, 70 completed 49 months of follow-up after placement of 2 iStents trabecular bypass stents and 1 iStent Supra in addition to postoperative travoprost. Mean medicated IOP was significantly reduced from 22.0 ± 3.1 mmHg preoperatively to 12.9 ± 0.9 mmHg postoperatively. Washout IOP demonstrated an over 30% reduction in diurnal IOP compared to pre-operative value. At the last follow up visit 97 and 98% of eyes achieved IOP ≤ 15 and ≤ 18 mmHg, respectively, on one medication. No eyes required additional glaucoma surgery although 10 eyes received subsequent cataract surgery and their IOP results were excluded from evaluation [32].

This study illustrates the potential for titrated surgery in some patients. Furthermore, in medical therapy, it is common to combine drugs that increase the aqueous outflow, either trabecular or uveoscleral, with drugs that decrease aqueous production. The results of this study support the hypothesis that a similar synergistic effect may be obtained with surgery. It is important to note that this was not reported in a peer-reviewed publication and hence caution is needed in interpreting the results.

MINIject

MINIject (iStar medical, USA) is supposed to address some of the drawbacks of previous suprachoroidal procedures/devices because of the characteristics of their proprietary material. The STAR material has been applied previously in the STARflo glaucoma implant: a suprachoroidal glaucoma drainage device designed for ab externo implantation that received CE marking in 2012 and which had no biocompatibility issues in clinical studies [33, 34]. The MINIject implant (Fig. 10) is made of the same STAR material, which is soft and flexible medical-grade silicone that conforms to the anatomic features of the eye. STAR material features innovative micropores characterized by hollow spheres arranged in a standardized network pattern. The soft material with a porous design encourages a natural flow speed and is intended to reduce the incidence of fibrosis and to minimize scarring, thus increasing implant durability. Studies on rabbits up to 26 weeks showed that the material is colonized by host cells, not preventing the aqueous humour drainage, thus avoiding long term IOP spikes due to fibrosis (in press).

The MINIject implant is 5 mm in length and has a rectangular cross-sectional shape measuring 1.1x0.6 mm with a green-colored ring at the proximal end, indicating the proper depth of placement (Fig. 10). The implant comes preloaded in a delivery tool that is used to enable the insertion of the implant into the supraciliary space of the eye via a minimally invasive ab interno procedure (Fig. 11). The release of the implant is different from both Cypass and iStent Supra. Because the implant is soft, it is held inside a protective sheath. The shaft is inserted through the anterior chamber towards the iridocorneal angle (Fig. 12). The sheath is advanced between the scleral spur and the ciliary body until the green ring is visible at the level of the scleral spur. When the position is correct, sliding the wheel retracts the protective sheath releasing the implant in place. When the middle of the green ring is positioned correctly at the level of the scleral spur, only 0.5 mm of the device remains in the anterior chamber reducing the potential for endothelial touch.

Fig. 10 The MINIject implant demonstrating the design of the STAR material with micropores technology. *(Courtesy of iStar medical, USA)*

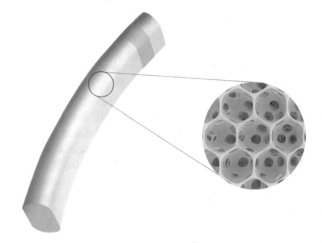

Fig. 11 The MINIject inserter. *(Courtesy of iStar medical, USA)*

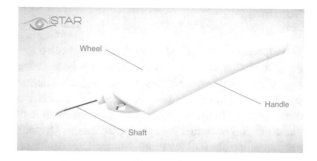

Fig. 12 Top: the sheath is introduced into the suprachoroidal space. Bottom: The sheath is retracted, leaving the implant in position *(Courtesy of iStar medical, USA)*

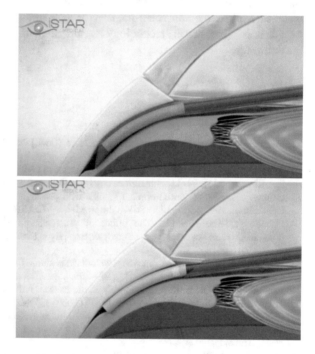

Denis et al. published the first in human result of the iStar implant in 26 POAG patients uncontrolled with one or more medications with 6 months follow up period [33]. Of the 25 eyes that had a successful implant, the mean IOP reduced from 23.3 ± 0.6 mmHg to 14.2 ± 0.9mmHfg. Medication was also reduced by 0.3 ± 0.7 drops. 87.5% of patient remained medication free at 6 months and 96% of patient achieved a 20% or more IOP reduction. No additional glaucoma surgery was required. Complications reported included hyphaema, IOP spikes and anterior chamber inflammation; all resolved without sequelae. Filli et all published their 12 months result demonstrating similar significant IOP reduction from 21.1 ± 7.3 mmHg preoperatively to 15.0 ± 25 mmHg postoperatively. However, 25% of patient failed requiring additional glaucoma surgery by 1 year [34].

Summary

The suprachoroidal space has most certainly been a fascinating yet frustrating space for glaucoma specialists. Much effort has been made to explore the potential of uveoscleral outflow with variable success. Its pharmacologic manipulation using prostaglandin analogues has been a significant landmark in glaucoma medication development. On the other hand, surgical exploration of the suprachoroidal space in glaucoma has been met with disappointments. Cyclodialysis cleft offers significant yet unpredictable IOP lowering. Supraciliary drainage devices have led to complications and failure due to fibrotic response. Nonetheless, continuous effort is being made to explore the suprachoroidal space as a treatment for glaucoma, and we would hope that newer technology would someday find an eagerly awaited breakthrough.

References

1. Nilsson SF. The uveoscleral outflow routes. Eye (Lond). 1997;11(Pt 2):149–54. https://doi.org/10.1038/eye.1997.43.PMID:9349404.
2. Johnson M, McLaren JW, Overby DR. Unconventional aqueous humor outflow: a review. Exp Eye Res. 2017;158:94–111. https://doi.org/10.1016/j.exer.2016.01.017.
3. Camras CB, Alm A. Initial clinical studies with prostaglandins and their analogues. Surv Ophthalmol. 1997;41(Suppl 2):S61–8. https://doi.org/10.1016/s0039-6257(97)80009-4.
4. Gabelt BT, Kaufman PL. The effect of prostaglandin F2 alpha on trabecular outflow facility in cynomolgus monkeys. Exp Eye Res. 1990;51(1):87–91. https://doi.org/10.1016/0014-4835(90)90174-s.
5. Gills JP, Paterson CA, Paterson ME. Cyclodialysis studied by manometric techniques in the monkey. Br J Ophthalmol. 1967;51(3):199–205. https://doi.org/10.1136/bjo.51.3.199.
6. Ioannidis AS, Barton K. Cyclodialysis cleft: causes and repair. Curr Opin Ophthalmol. 2010;21(2):150–4. https://doi.org/10.1097/ICU.0b013e3283366a4d.
7. González-Martín-Moro J, Contreras-Martín I, Muñoz-Negrete FJ, Gómez-Sanz F, Zarallo-Gallardo J. Cyclodialysis: an update. Int Ophthalmol. 2017;37(2):441–57. https://doi.org/10.1007/s10792-016-0282-8.
8. Jing Q, Chen J, Chen J, Tang Y, Lu Y, Jiang Y. Cionni-modified capsular tension ring for surgical repair of cyclodialysis after trabeculectomy: a case report. BMC Ophthalmol. 2017;17(1):196. https://doi.org/10.1186/s12886-017-0582-4.
9. Mardelli PG. Closure of persistent cyclodialysis cleft using the haptics of the intraocular lens. Am J Ophthalmol. 2006;142(4):676–8. https://doi.org/10.1016/j.ajo.2006.05.027.
10. Helbig H, Foerster MH. Management of hypotonous cyclodialysis with pars plana vitrectomy, gas tamponade, and cryotherapy. Ophthalmic Surg Lasers. 1996;27(3):188–91.
11. Böke H. Zur Geschichte der Zyklodialyse. In memoriam Leopold Heine 1870-1940 [History of cyclodialysis. In memory of Leopold Heine 1870-1940]. Klin Monatsbl Augenheilkd. 1990;197(4):340–8. https://doi.org/10.1055/s-2008-1046291.
12. Aviner Z. Modified Krasnov's iridocycloretraction for aphakic glaucoma. Ann Ophthalmol. 1975;7(6):859–61.
13. Barkan O, Boyle SF, Maisler S. On the surgery of glaucoma: mode of action of cyclodialysis. Cal West Med. 1936;44(1):12–6.

14. Flieringa HJ. Cyclodialysis combined with posterior trephining. Br J Ophthalmol. 1952;36(9):518–9. https://doi.org/10.1136/bjo.36.9.518.
15. Dada T, Sharma R, Sinha G, Angmo D, Temkar S. Cyclodialysis-enhanced trabeculectomy with triple ologen implantation. Eur J Ophthalmol. 2016;26(1):95–7. https://doi.org/10.5301/ejo.5000633.
16. Gills JP. Cyclodialysis implants in human eyes. Am J Ophthalmol. 1966;61(5 Pt 1):841–6. https://doi.org/10.1016/0002-9394(66)90922-6.
17. Gills JP Jr, Paterson CA, Paterson ME. Mode of action of cyclodialysis implants in man. Investig Ophthalmol. 1967;6(2):141–4.
18. Nesterov AP, Kolesnikova LN. Implantation of a scleral strip into the supraciliary space and cyclodialysis in glaucoma. Acta Ophthalmol. 1978;56(5):697–704. https://doi.org/10.1111/j.1755-3768.1978.tb06633.x.
19. Ozdamar A, Aras C, Karacorlu M. Suprachoroidal seton implantation in refractory glaucoma: a novel surgical technique. J Glaucoma. 2003;12(4):354–9. https://doi.org/10.1097/00061198-200308000-00010.
20. Melamed S, Ben Simon GJ, Goldenfeld M, Simon G. Efficacy and safety of gold micro shunt implantation to the supraciliary space in patients with glaucoma: a pilot study. Arch Ophthalmol. 2009;127(3):264–9. https://doi.org/10.1001/archophthalmol.2008.611.
21. Figus M, Lazzeri S, Fogagnolo P, Iester M, Martinelli P, Nardi M. Supraciliary shunt in refractory glaucoma. Br J Ophthalmol. 2011;95(11):1537–41. https://doi.org/10.1136/bjophthalmol-2011-300308.
22. Skaat A, Sagiv O, Kinori M, Ben Simon GJ, Goldenfeld M, Melamed S. Gold micro-shunt implants versus Ahmed glaucoma valve: long-term outcomes of a prospective randomized clinical trial. J Glaucoma. 2016;25(2):155–61. https://doi.org/10.1097/IJG.0000000000000175.
23. Hueber A, Roters S, Jordan JF, Konen W. Retrospective analysis of the success and safety of Gold Micro Shunt Implantation in glaucoma. BMC Ophthalmol. 2013;13:35. https://doi.org/10.1186/1471-2415-13-35.
24. Figus M, Posarelli C, Passani A, et al. The supraciliary space as a suitable pathway for glaucoma surgery: Ho-hum or home run? Surv Ophthalmol. 2017;62(6):828–37. https://doi.org/10.1016/j.survophthal.2017.05.002.
25. Rękas M, Pawlik B, Grala B, Kozłowski W. Clinical and morphological evaluation of gold micro shunt after unsuccessful surgical treatment of patients with primary open-angle glaucoma. Eye (Lond). 2013;27(10):1214–7. https://doi.org/10.1038/eye.2013.154.
26. Höh H, Grisanti S, Grisanti S, Rau M, Ianchulev S. Two-year clinical experience with the CyPass micro-stent: safety and surgical outcomes of a novel supraciliary micro-stent. Klin Monatsbl Augenheilkd. 2014;231(4):377–81. https://doi.org/10.1055/s-0034-1368214.
27. Vold S, Ahmed II, Craven ER, et al. Two-year COMPASS trial results: supraciliary microstenting with phacoemulsification in patients with open-angle glaucoma and cataracts. Ophthalmology. 2016;123(10):2103–12. https://doi.org/10.1016/j.ophtha.2016.06.032.
28. García-Feijoo J, Rau M, Grisanti S, et al. Supraciliary micro-stent implantation for open-angle glaucoma failing topical therapy: 1-year results of a multicenter study. Am J Ophthalmol. 2015;159(6):1075–1081.e1. https://doi.org/10.1016/j.ajo.2015.02.018.
29. https://www.fda.gov/medical-devices/medical-device-recalls/alcon-research-ltd-recalls-cypassr-micro-stent-systems-due-risk-endothelial-cell-loss
30. Manasses DT, Au L. The new era of glaucoma micro-stent surgery. Ophthalmol Ther. 2016;5:135–46.
31. Junemann A. Twelve-month outcomes following ab interno implantation of suprachoroidal stent and postoperative administration of travoprost to treat open-angle glaucoma. Amsterdam, Netherlands: 31st Congress of the European Society of Cataract and Refractive Surgeons; Oct, 2013.
32. Myers JS, Masood I, Hornbeak DM, Belda JI, Auffarth G, Jünemann A, Giamporcaro JE, Martinez-de-la-Casa JM, Ahmed IIK, Voskanyan L, Katz LJ. Prospective evaluation of two

Istent® trabecular stents, one Istent Supra® suprachoroidal stent, and postoperative prostaglandin in refractory glaucoma: 4-year outcomes. Adv Ther. 2018 Mar;35(3):395–407.

33. Denis P, Hirneiß C, Reddy KS, Kamarthy A, Calvo E, Hussain Z, Ahmed IIK. A first-in-human study of the efficacy and safety of MINIject in patients with medically uncontrolled open-angle glaucoma (STAR-I). Ophthalmol Glaucoma. 2019;2:290–7.

34. Fili S, Wolfelschneider P, Kohlhaas M. The STARflo glaucoma implant: preliminary 12 months results. Graefes Arch Clin Exp Ophthalmol. 2018;256(4):773e781.

Suprachoroidal Buckling for Peripheral Retinal Breaks

Peter Szurman

Introduction

Rhegmatogenous retinal detachment is the most important retinal surgical emergency with an incidence of approximately 1:10,000 per year or 1:300 over the entire life span [1]. This results in annual primary retinal detachment surgery in about 8000 cases in Germany [2] and 28,000 cases in the US [3].

Since Jules Gonin, the treatment of retinal detachment has been based on the principle of identification and closure of a causative retinal tear [4]. Both buckling surgery and vitrectomy are established procedures for this purpose. As different as the surgical approaches may appear at first glance, both techniques follow the principle of approximation and fixation presented by Custodis in 1953 [5]. Either the approximation is done externally by suturing a scleral buckle and fixation with cryopexy, or internally by vitrectomy with approximation by endotamponade and fixation by laser retinopexy (Table 1). Although we have experienced continuous technical refinements in recent years, the basic principle has remained unchanged.

Both techniques have their advantages and disadvantages: The main advantage of buckling surgery is the lens-sparing effect. However, classical buckling surgery is technically obsolete, as the use of low-detail indirect ophthalmoscopy, poor indirect illumination and more invasive cryopexy are limiting [6]. It has not benefited from the technological advances that modern vitrectomy has experienced in recent years. Further disadvantages of scleral buckling are the large-area peritomy, the poor accessibility of retinal tears located under the muscles and the risk of postoperative diplopia [7] or buckle migration. Due to the technical superiority of

P. Szurman (✉)
Eye Clinic Sulzbach, Knappschaft Hospital Saar, Sulzbach, Germany

Klaus Heimann Eye Research Institute, Sulzbach, Germany
e-mail: Peter.Szurman@kksaar.de

Table 1 Principle of approximation and fixation in retinal detachment surgery

	Approximation	Fixation
Vitrectomy	Hydrophobic tamponade	Laserpexy
Buckling surgery	Scleral buckle or encircling band	Cryopexy
Suprachoroidal hydrogel buckle	Suprachoroidal hydrogel	Laserpexy (or Cryo)

vitrectomy and the ever-decreasing range of training, classical buckle surgery is increasingly being ousted from clinical routine [8].

Conversely, vitrectomy has benefited from the continuous technical refinement in recent years [9–11]. In particular, high-resolution visualisation with wide-angle viewing systems, high magnification on modern microscopes, effective endoillumination and gentle endolaser coagulation have made this technique more effective and safer [12, 13]. The introduction of trocar-guided surgery supports the increasingly minimally invasive character of modern vitrectomy. However, vitrectomy has the major disadvantage of progressive cataract development [14] and tamponade-associated problems such as temporary visual loss, intraocular pressure fluctuations [15] or the need for a second intervention when using non-resorbable tamponades.

Suprachoroidal Hydrogel Buckle

Combining the Best of Both Worlds

The suprachoroidal hydrogel buckle combines the best of both worlds: The advantages of lens-sparing buckling surgery with targeted sealing of the retinal break but at the same time the use of modern ophthalmic surgical techniques with wide-angle visualisation on the operating microscope, endoillumination and laser retinopexy.

It is also mandatory for such a minimally invasive technique that it can be performed easily and quickly, does not require a large-area peritomy of the conjunctiva and avoids scleral buckle-associated problems. In particular, retinal breaks in the area of the eye muscles should be easily accessible to avoid diplopia.

In this overview, we show the wide range of applications of the minimally invasive suprachoroidal hydrogel buckle, which combines all these advantages and for the first time allows to combine classical buckling surgery with the modern technological achievements of vitrectomy. We also present the different properties and biocompatibility of the hydrogel variants already used for the suprachoroidal hydrogel buckle.

The Rationale of Suprachoroidal Hydrogel Buckle

The original variants of buckling surgery were all based on an episcleral approach. The basic principle of the suprachoroidal hydrogel buckle is that the indenting effect is not caused by an episcleral buckle, but by injecting a hydrogel through a small

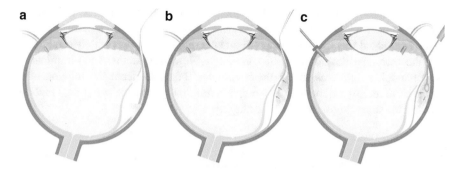

Fig. 1 Schematic drawing of suprachoroidal buckling. The suprachoroidal catheter is advanced underneath the retinal tear (*A*). By injecting viscoelastic into the suprachoroidal space, the retinal tear is sealed by a dome-shaped choroid displacement (*B*). Alternatively, the entire process can be performed with an olive tip cannula (*C*). The images illustrate either a stand-alone procedure with 27 g chandelier light (*A* + *B*) or a combined procedure with trocar-guided endoillumination and infusion (*C*)

transscleral incision into the suprachoroidal space (Fig. 1). Only the choroid and the retinal pigment epithelium are approximated to the retina by the hydrogel, but not the sclera. It reduces vitreous traction and diminishes the flux of vitreous fluid through retinal tears, thus promoting reposition of the retina to the retinal pigment epithelium (RPE). Achieving this goal through the suprachoroidal space instead of scleral indentation avoids some of the difficulties associated with episcleral buckles.

Historical Development

There have been numerous pioneering studies testing the principle of a suprachoroidal buckling procedure for the minimally invasive treatment of retinal detachment. By using fillers based on air [16], gelatin [17], fibrin [18, 19], fat [20] or urethane polymer [21] they could indent the choroid and create a suprachoroidal buckling effect to close the tears.

However, the decisive breakthrough was achieved by the groups of Poole and Mittl, who presented a novel, minimally invasive technique by suprachoroidal injection of viscoelastic. Poole and Sudarsky introduced a new suprachoroidal buckling technique using a blunt 27-gauge needle and slowly injecting 0.2–0.8 ml 1% sodium hyaluronate (Healon®) posteriorly into the suprachoroidal space to separate choroid from sclera in 1986. In a study with 14 patients, they reported a sufficient buckling effect for up to 2 weeks and achieved successful reattachment in all cases [22]. Mittl und Tiwari compared both non-crosslinked and cross-linked sodium hyaluronate (1 and 2%) and observed no significant differences between buckles created. They described the buckling effect as short-lived, but sodium hyaluronate survived in the suprachoroidal space up to 10–14 days or more. The authors concluded that Internal buckling of the choroid might prove to be a viable adjunct or alternative to conventional buckling procedures [23].

Despite these hopeful studies, the principle initially could not prevail. This was not due to the surgical technique or the available hydrogels but was somewhat due to the fact that at that time classical scleral buckling surgery was widely established and the technical development of wide-angle viewing systems, endoillumination and chandelier light was still in the beginning. Today, the technical refinement of modern vitrectomy offers us a wide range of minimally invasive equipment that can be used for suprachoroidal buckling surgery.

Working in the Suprachoroidal Space

Another reason was that many ophthalmic surgeons at that time had respectful fear for the choroid. They were worried that manipulation in the suprachoroidal space would involve a high risk of complications. This concern has partly disappeared today, as choroid manipulation has become routine in various operations.

In non-penetrating glaucoma surgery, for example in modified canaloplasty with suprachoroidal drainage, the suprachoroidal space is routinely exposed, widened extensively with viscoelastic, and the choroid is buckled up with a voluminous collagen sponge. Large studies with 1000 patients were able to show that there are no choroid-associated complications, in particular, no expulsive hemorrhage [24–26].

Also, studies on choroidal patch translocation in AMD surgery have shown that parts of the choroid can be excised, coagulated and relocated as a free graft without choroid-associated complications [27, 28].

Milestones in Technical Refinement

A significant milestone in 2010 was the development of a microcatheter designed for drug application into the suprachoroidal space (iTrack 400, iScience). This catheter is easy to introduce via a small sclerotomy and allows free manoeuvring within the suprachoroidal space and controlling target structures. Studies showed a controlled placement of both drugs for retinal diseases [29] and viscoelastic for suprachoroidal buckling of retinal breaks [30].

However, the broad popularisation of the suprachoroidal buckle was achieved by El-Rayes in 2013, who made a comprehensive refinement of the surgical technique and described different variants in detail. He developed a specially designed 450 mm catheter for macular buckling and posterior breaks [31], and an Olive tip cannula for suprachoroidal buckling of peripheral breaks (both MedOne Surgical, Sarasota, FL) [32]. A detailed summary of surgical techniques and equipment can be found in an excellent book review [33].

Our safety data from rabbit experiments showed that the suprachoroidal space is a safe location for a hydrogel buckle for both non-crosslinked and cross-linked viscoelastic (Healaflow®, Aptissen, Genf, Schweiz). Neither clinical signs of cataract formation or intraocular inflammation nor histological retinotoxicity were detected (Fig. 2) [30].

With the withdrawal of classical buckle surgery from clinical routine as well as technical improvements and more stable hydrogels, the suprachoroidal hydrogel buckle has become increasingly established and is used by more surgeons as a third, equivalent procedure for the treatment of rhegmatogenous ablation. In the meantime, larger studies with long-term results have been published, reporting a high success rate of 92%–100% (Table 2) [30, 34–35].

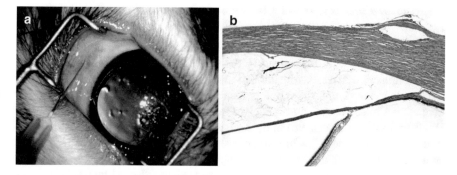

Fig. 2 Intraoperative photography (**a**) of suprachoroidal buckling in rabbit eyes using cross-linked hydrogel (Healaflow®) and histology after 2 weeks (**b**)

Table 2 Overview of the results from patient studies on suprachoroidal buckling for peripheral retinal breaks

Authors	No. of patients	Success rate	Technique
Poole and Sudarsky, (1984) [22]	14	100%	Blunt 27 g cannula Healon® Combined with scleral buckle (86%)
Szurman et al. (2016) [30]	21	95%	Olive tip cannula (90%)—Catheter (10%) Combined (71%)—Stand-alone (29%) Healon® (67%)—Healaflow® (33%) Slit lamp laser postop. (100%)
El Rayes et al. (2017) [34]	41	93%	Olive tip cannula Stand-alone (88%)—Combined (12%) Restylane® (63%)—Healon 5® (37%) Cryo (90%)—Indirect laser (10%)
Mikhail et al. (2017) [35]	62	92%	Catheter Stand-alone (76%)—Combined (24%) Healon 5® (89%)—Healon GV® (8%)—Restylane® (3%) Cryo (61%)—Indirect laser (39%)

Surgical Technique

Two Surgical Approaches to Suprachoroidal Buckling Surgery

The suprachoroidal hydrogel buckle can either be used additively in combination with a vitrectomy or as a stand-alone procedure [30, 34–35]. As a combined procedure, it is mainly used to support inferior breaks during vitrectomy by adding a transient buckling effect in order to solve a difficult tamponade situation. As a stand-alone procedure, it replaces the classic buckling surgery.

Suprachoroidal Hydrogel Buckle Combined with Vitrectomy

In the combined procedure, a standard 3-port vitrectomy with transconjunctival 23-gauge trocars is performed using the usual wide-angle viewing system and endoillumination. After identification of the causative break ab interno, the vitreous traction is relieved, and the retina is reattached with perfluorocarbon liquid. The conjunctiva in the tear region is incised, and a small radial sclerotomy of 2 mm length and a 4 mm distance from the limbus is performed until the underlying choroid is identified. Under low infusion pressure, the choroid can be pushed back with some viscoelastic (Healon®) to create a suprachoroidal cavity under the sclerotomy with sufficient safety distance from the choroid. Then either a blunt olive tip cannula or a microcatheter can be advanced in the suprachoroidal space. Under direct visualisation with the wide-angle viewing system and endoillumination cannula or catheter is manoeuvred under the break. By injecting the hydrogel into the suprachoroidal space, a suprachoroidal buckle of variable height and width can be created until the break is sufficiently sealed. In the case of several tears, the hydrogel can be distributed up to 120° by moving the cannula, creating a buckling effect parallel to the limbus. The fixation can be performed as usual with endolaser coagulation. At the end of the vitrectomy, an internal tamponade can be used (Fig. 3).

The suprachoroidal hydrogel buckle combined with vitrectomy is recommended whenever a supportive buckling effect, usually inferiorly, is necessary during vitrectomy. This usually occurs in PVR surgery or with multiple, inferior breaks with thinned retina and a relevant risk of re-detachment under gas or oil. In such complicated situations with extensive traction or retinal shortening, an additive encircling or limbus parallel buckle can provide relief. In the age of transconjunctival trocar-guided vitrectomy, however, many surgeons refrain from applying an additional encircling band because this is time-consuming and shows significantly more irritation postoperatively than a vitrectomy without [36, 37].

Instead, with this new technique, it can be decided at any time point of vitrectomy to create an additional indenting effect at the vitreous base by means of a hydrogel buckle with minimal time and only minor conjunctival preparation.

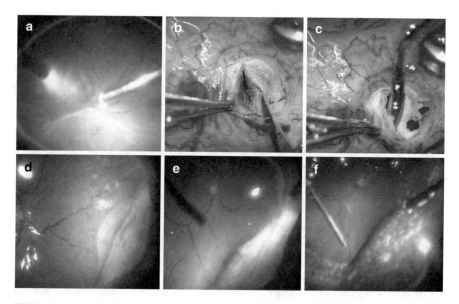

Fig. 3 Combined suprachoroidal buckle with vitrectomy. PVR-retinal detachment with multiple breaks (**a**). A scleral incision with identification of the choroid (**b**). Cannulation of the suprachoroidal space using an olive tip cannula (**c**). Advancing underneath the retinal break under direct visualisation ab interno (**d**). A buckle is created and can be adjusted to the individual situation (**e**). Endophotocoagulation of well-supported retinal breaks (**f**)

In our study, we used the hydrogel buckle mainly as a combined procedure (71%), especially in vitrectomy cases where intraoperatively an unfavourable position of the breaks was evident, and an additional buckling effect seemed advantageous [30]. Other research groups use the combined procedure less frequently (12–20%), as they prefer the stand-alone procedure, but also with a high success rate [34, 35].

A further advantage is the use of lighter tamponade: silicone oil can often be replaced by gas or air or no tamponade. In our study cohort, patients received only SF6 gas (40%), air (27%) or no tamponade (30% BSS) despite a complex initial situation with inferior breaks and PVR [30].

Suprachoroidal Hydrogel Buckle as a Stand-Alone Procedure

As a replacement for classical buckle surgery, the suprachoroidal hydrogel buckle can also be used as a stand-alone procedure without vitrectomy. Only an endoillumination with 27 g chandelier light (Twin-Light, DORC) is introduced. Thus, identification of retinal breaks can be performed under the microscope ab interno via the usual wide-angle viewing system. A vitrectomy is not performed.

The placement of the 27 g chandelier endoillumination should be applied oppo-site to the preoperatively identified breaks ensuring uniform light distribution. The conjunctiva is then incised in the tear quadrant and a small radial sclerotomy of approx. 2 mm length at 4 mm distance from the limbus is prepared until the underly-ing choroid is identified. A subsequent paracentesis achieves hypotony—analogous to scleral buckling surgery—to avoid prolapse or injury of the choroid. The choroid is pushed back with viscoelastic (Healon®) to create a suprachoroidal cavity under the sclerotomy with sufficient safety distance to the choroid. In the case of bullous retinal detachment, some authors perform subretinal drainage [34, 35], while we refrain from doing so for safety reasons [30].

Subsequently, the suprachoroidal space is probed, and the injection cannula is advanced. The suprachoroidal buckling effect is generated in a controlled manner under direct visualisation with wide-angle viewing system and chandelier light. Retinopexy is performed either with cryopexy prior to injection or, better, on the first postoperative day with laser photocoagulation at the slit lamp (Fig. 4).

In contrast to the combined procedure, the intraoperative pressure should be—analogous to the scleral buckling surgery—observed closely. Before opening the suprachoroidal space, paracentesis of the anterior chamber should be performed to relieve pressure. The amount of hydrogel injected should also be limited to a maxi-mum of 0.8 ml. Thus, large hydrogel buckles parallel to the limbus are not possible

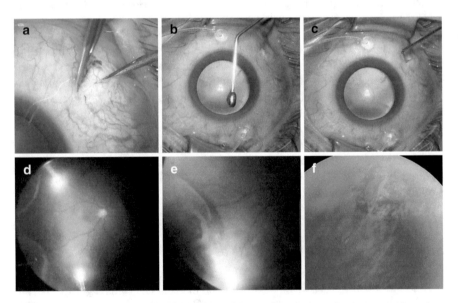

Fig. 4 Suprachoroidal buckle as a stand-alone procedure. A scleral incision with a minimal con-junctival opening (**a**). Olive tip cannula and two chandelier lights (TwinLight, DORC) (**b**). Introducing the cannula underneath the choroid (**c**). Identification of the retinal break under direct visualisation ab interno using the olive tip for choroidal indentation (**d**). A buckle is created and can be adjusted to the individual situation (**e**). Stable scarring 8 weeks after photocoagulation performed at the first postoperative day using slit lamp laser (**f**)

in the stand-alone procedure. High pressure can also lead to a prolapse and incarceration of the vitreous into the sclerotomy of the chandelier light. The sclerotomy is sutured with vicryl 8–0.

The suprachoroidal hydrogel buckle as a stand-alone procedure is ideally suited for classic single-break surgery. It includes all the advantages of scleral buckling surgery, especially the lens sparing effect, but is much less invasive and more time-efficient. In addition, direct visualisation of retinal holes under the operating microscope with wide-angle magnifying system and endo-light is clearly superior to indirect ophthalmoscopy. A further advantage is that retinal tears under the eye muscles are also easily accessible. Thus, postoperative diplopia is avoided.

The suprachoroidal hydrogel buckle corresponds to a significant technical modernisation of classical buckle surgery and is suitable to replace it in uncomplicated retinal detachment surgery. A live surgery video can be found at https://youtu.be/QcUmzPXduT0.

Catheter or Cannula?

Catheter

The use of catheters helps in targeting posteriorly located pathologies such as myopic vitreomacular interface problems or posteriorly located retinal breaks. It is particularly suitable for creating macular buckles to treat myopic macular holes (see Chapter "Suprachoroidal Buckling for Myopic Macular Holes") [38]. The catheter must have a sufficiently large lumen to apply all available hydrogels (cross-linked or non-crosslinked). Two catheter systems have been available:

In 2010, a novel microcatheter was introduced specially designed for drug application into the suprachoroidal space (iTrack 400, iScience). This variation of the normal iTrack 250 for canaloplasty has an extended lumen and allows atraumatic probing of the suprachoroidal space under visual guidance of the illuminated tip with direct visualisation of position. An experimental animal study in 93 pigs and monkeys could show that suprachoroidal catheterisation and the controlled application of drugs in the suprachoroidal space is possible [29]. In a larger patient cohort we could show that this catheter is also suitable for the application of both non-crosslinked HA (Healon®) and cross-linked HA (Healaflow®) into the suprachoroidal space and thereby sealing peripheral breaks by a suprachoroidal hydrogel buckle (Fig. 5) [30].

In 2013, El-Rayes and Oshima introduced a specially designed, illuminated, 450 µm wide, flex-tip catheter (patent pending; MedOne Surgical, Sarasota, FL) for suprachoroidal buckling [31]. This catheter has a dual injection illumination capability. It can be connected to a regular light source that illuminates a 31-gauge light fibre when placed in the suprachoroidal space. The other end of the Y connector on the catheter is connected to high-pressure tubing to deliver the filler, which forms

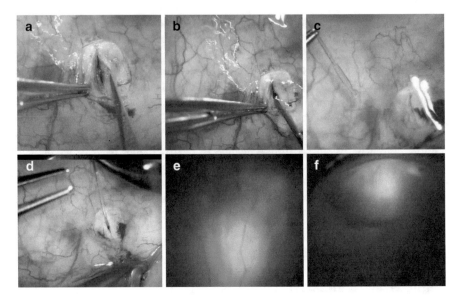

Fig. 5 Catheter-guided suprachoroidal buckling. A scleral incision with identification of the choroid (**a**). The choroid is pushed back with Healon® to create a safe cavity for cannulation (**b**). Microcatheter for suprachoroidal drug application with illuminated tip (iTrack 400, iScience) (**c**). Introduction of the catheter into the suprachoroidal space (**d**). Advancing the catheter under direct visualisation ab interno (**e**). A buckle is created and can be adjusted to the individual situation (**f**). Laserpexy will be performed the day after surgery

the choroidal dome. In a feasibility study, the authors could show that long-lasting, cross-linked HA fillers could be applied (Restylane Perlane; Q-Med, Uppsala, Sweden). In a larger study, suprachoroidal indentation was achieved through the introduction of Healon 5 (89%), Healon GV (8%) or Restylane-Perlane (3%) with a success rate of 92% [35].

The main advantage of catheter-guided buckling is the free navigation in the suprachoroidal space. Posteriorly located breaks can be targeted irrelevant to the anterior location of the sclerotomy. It also allows for targeting multiple breaks at different positions via one entry site. The illuminated tip of the catheter facilitates the exact positioning and placement of the filler underneath the break.

Olive Tip Cannula

As an alternative, El Rayes and Eborgy introduced in 2013 a single-use curved suprachoroidal cannula (MedOne Surgical) specially designed for suprachoroidal buckling [32]. The cannula is not illuminated, but the advantage of the blunt olive tip is that it acts as a choroidal depressor to locate the retinal break under direct visualisation with the operating microscope using wide angle viewing system and endoillumination. After correct placement exactly underneath the tear, the viscoelastic is injected, creating a controlled suprachoroidal buckle effect.

In their feasibility study, they injected Restylane, which is a high purity cross-linked hyaluronic acid gel and could create an appropriate dome-shaped choroidal indentation. In a larger study with 41 patients, they achieved a success rate of 92% by using this technique [34].

As a simple alternative, we either use a disposable curved olive tip cannula (Olive tip cannula, BVI, Waltham, MA) or a reusable Gills-Welsh Olive tip cannula for cortex aspiration (Gills-Welsh Olive Tip 25-g Cannula, MSI, Phoenixville, PA). We connect it to a short extension tube allowing the nurse to inject the hydrogel in a controlled manner, while the surgeon manoeuvres the cannula. Alternatively, a new prototype may facilitate handling (Fig. 6).

In our study with 21 patients, we could show the viability for both non-crosslinked HA (Healon®) and cross-linked HA (Healaflow®) through this cannula and success-ful suprachoroidal buckling without any choroidal complications [30].

The main advantage of using a cannula instead of a catheter is that it can be used as a gentle choroidal depressor for identifying the break. The blunt olive tip avoids harming the choroid during this manipulation. Furthermore, the cannula shows superior results in the treatment of retinal holes compared to the catheter. By turning the curved cannula, the surgeon can reach two clock hours on either side of the entry point, so that a circumferential buckle effect of about four clock hours is possible. Other authors were able to reach up to 180° via one entry site [34]. Therefore, in our clinic, we only use the choroidal depressor cannula instead of the catheter.

The disadvantage of the cannula is its restriction to peripheral pathology only. Posterior breaks, especially in the post-equatorial region, are not accessible. Also, the region of the vortex veins must be avoided. Finally, the cannula may potentially bear a higher risk of harming the choroid than the catheter due to the manipulation during the choroidal depression. One study reported two localised suprachoroidal haemorrhages at the entry site, which were observed and resolved without further intervention [34].

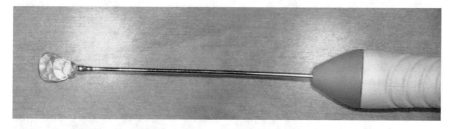

Fig. 6 A prototype of choroidal indentor with an olive tip designed for suprachoroidal buckling

Laser or Cryo Retinopexy

In the combined surgical technique, retinopexy can be performed as usual with an endolaser, since the hydrogel under the choroid does not influence the laser's reaction between the retinal pigment epithelium and the retina. In contrast, the stand-alone procedure offers several possibilities for retinopexy:

El-Rayes used cryotherapy in 90% of cases, whereas indirect laser was used to create chorioretinal adhesion in 10% of cases [34]. Cryotherapy was applied before the buckle, whereas laser was applied after the buckle using indirect ophthalmoscopy. In the largest to date study, Mikhail et al. used cryopexy and indirect laser retinopexy in equal parts [35].

In our study, we proposed a different technique for retinopexy [30]. In our opinion, cryopexy weakens the tissue and bears the risk of choroidal injury, especially during the choroidal indentation. Indirect binocular ophthalmoscope (BIO) laser retinopexy is also not a contemporary alternative. It is significantly gentler and more controlled if the laser photocoagulation is performed on the first postoperative day with a conventional argon/diode laser at the slit lamp. Since the break is well buckled and there is no intraocular inflammation, this is easily performed. In some cases, however, complete resorption of the subretinal fluid must be awaited to achieve sufficiently strong laser effects (Fig. 7).

Biocompatibility and Resorption Time of the Different Hydrogels

The important parameter is the appropriate choice of viscoelastic substance to be injected. Poole demanded that the ideal material for a temporary suprachoroidal buckle should have the following properties: be injectable through a small-gauge needle, yet viscous enough to maintain the shape and position of the suprachoroidal

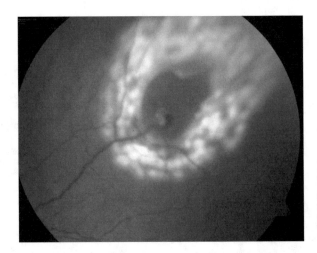

Fig. 7 Laserpexy after suprachoroidal buckling (without vitrectomy) performed two days postoperatively. Perfect insight without any inflammation, the edges of the break are attached and buckled up. Hence laser retinopexy can easily be performed

implant; remain in the suprachoroidal space long enough for the formation of an adequate chorioretinal scar (at least 7–10 days); be immunologically inert; provoke no inflammation, and reabsorb entirely without sequelae [22].

Nowadays, we have a broad range of non-crosslinked and cross-linked fillers (Fig. 8) that can be used to create the desired choroidal indentation effect. Hyaluronic acid can be modified by either molecular weight or cross-linking to create longer resistance to resorption (Fig. 9, Table 3).

The results of the available studies suggest that a tamponade time of 1 week may be sufficient. The buckling effect relieves vitreoretinal traction, and the chorioretinal adhesion around the retinal break is significantly increased 24 h after laser coagulation. After 3 days it is already three times more adherent than the normal retina [39].

A short-term buckling effect with non-crosslinked hydrogel thus appears to be sufficient for most situations according to the concurring study results. However,

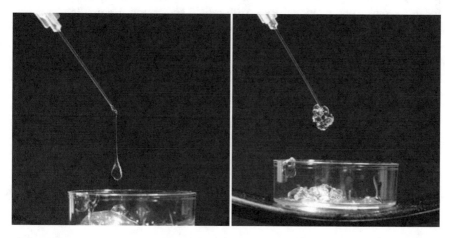

Fig. 8 Different viscosity and rheological characteristics of non-crosslinked (left, Healon®) and cross-linked (right, Healaflow®) hyaluronic acid viscoelastic hydrogel

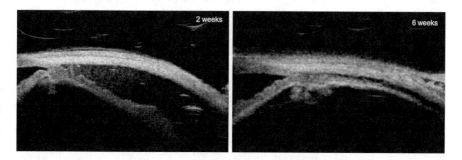

Fig. 9 50 MHz ultrasound biomicroscopy after suprachoroidal buckling using cross-linked Healaflow®

Table 3 Overview of possible viscoelastic candidates, including approval status and retention time in the suprachoroidal space

Product		Approval	x-linked	Visible buckling effect
Healon® Abbott medical optics, USA	10 mg/mL	Intraocular use	No	5–10 days [22, 30]
Healon GV® Abbott Medical Optics, USA	14 mg/ml	Intraocular use	No	7–8 days [30, 35]
Healon 5® Abbott Medical Optics, USA	23 mg/ml	Intraocular use	No	3 weeks [35]
Healaflow® Aptissen, Switzerland	22.5 mg/ml	Glaucoma surgery	x-linked	5–8 weeks [30]
Restylane Perlane® Galderma, Switzerland	20 mg/ml	Dermal filler	x-linked	4 months [34, 35]

depending on the individual situation, the surgeon can deliberately choose a more prolonged buckling effect with a cross-linked filler. The most important indication for this seems to be tractional PVR with retinal shortening. Here, a longer-acting support of the peripheral retina over several months may be necessary, which can only be achieved with cross-linked fillers.

In addition, biocompatibility is an ongoing issue. The biocompatibility of non-crosslinked HA viscoelastic is well known from cataract surgery [40]. Although most of the fillers used are approved for ophthalmic use, the specific biocompatibility in the suprachoroidal space has not yet been finally clarified for all potential viscoelastic candidates. The available human studies indicate favourable biocompatibility. Histological data from rabbit eyes are available for Healon®, Healon GV® and Healaflow® [30].

Complications and the Learning Curve

Besides re-detachment, haemorrhage is the most common complication. In our study only in one case a slight bleeding in the sclerotomy area, but not intraocularly, was observed, which stopped spontaneously. However, a recent study shows that the risk of haemorrhagic complications is increased explicitly during the learning curve phase [41]. The authors found localised subretinal haemorrhages in 6 of 23 eyes that were mostly self-limited and did not affect final visual outcome. Only one case experienced severe visual loss. All haemorrhages were inferior, adjacent to the site of the tear, and occurred during external fluid drainage or injection of the viscoelastic material or during fluid- air exchange. Other complications, especially ischaemic choroidal changes or hyperpigmentation, were not observed.

Of interest, all six complications occurred during the surgical learning curve, as they were part of the first ten consecutive eyes that underwent suprachoroidal buckling. No complications occurred in the following 13 cases. This underlines the importance of careful manipulation and conscientious guidance during the learning curve.

Conclusion

The suprachoroidal placement of a hydrogel buckle appears to be a simple, fast and effective therapy for retinal detachment as reported by Poole and El-Rayes. It combines the advantages of both worlds and can be performed either in combination with a vitrectomy or as a stand-alone procedure. With the combined procedure, it is possible to easily and quickly create an additional buckle in the area of increased traction. In vitrectomy procedures for retinal detachment with inferior breaks, this can possibly prevent an oil tamponade and thus a revisional operation. The suprachoroidal buckle is also elegant as a stand-alone procedure, since it incorporates all the advantages of classic scleral buckle surgery, especially the lens-preserving effect, while at the same time makes use of modern vitrectomy techniques with direct visualisation under a wide-angle viewing system and gentle laser coagulation. In addition to the minimally invasive character and the resorption of the temporary buckle, the good access to retinal tears, including those under the extraocular recti muscles, is of great advantage as this avoids ocular motility disorders and diplopia. It can be used for the treatment of single or multiple tears. In our opinion, the avoidance of cryopexy and the use of gentle laser photocoagulation on the first postoperative day at the slit lamp is preferable. Overall, the studies show a low complication rate. We evaluate the suprachoroidal hydrogel buckle as a sustainable procedure that is increasingly establishing itself as a third, equivalent method for treating retinal detachment.

References

1. Haimann MH, Burton TC, Brown CK. Epidemiology of retinal detachment. Arch Ophthalmol. 1982;100:289–92.
2. Feltgen N, Walter P. Rhegmatogenous retinal detachment--an ophthalmologic emergency. Dtsch Arztebl Int. 2014;111:12–21.
3. Subramanian ML, Topping TM. Controversies in the management of primary retinal detachments. Int Ophthalmol Clin. 2004;44:103–14.
4. Gonin J. Le traitement de décollement rétinien. Ann Oculist. 1921;158
5. Custodis E. Bedeutet die Plombenaufnaehung auf die Sklera einen Fortschritt in der operativen Behandlung der Netzhautablösung. Ber Dtsch Ophthalmol Ges. 1953;58:102.
6. Abdullah AS, Jan S, Qureshi MS, Khan MT, Khan MD. Complications of conventional scleral buckling occuring during and after treatment of rhegmatogenous retinal detachment. J Coll Physicians Surg Pakistan. 2010;5:321–6.
7. Chaudhry NL, Durnian JM. Post-vitreoretinal surgery strabismus - a review. Strabismus. 2012;20:26–30.
8. Ah-Fat FG, Sharma MC, Majid M, McGalliard JN, Wong D. Trends in vitreoretinal surgery at a tertiary referral centre: 1987 to 1996. Br J Ophthalmol. 1999;83:396–8.
9. Eckardt C. Transconjunctival sutureless 23-gauge vitrectomy. Retina. 2005;25:208–11.
10. Ibarra MS, Hermel M, Prenner JL, Hassan TS. Longer-term outcomes of transconjunctival sutureless 25-gauge vitrectomy. Am J Ophthalmol. 2005;139:831–6.
11. Ghasemi Falavarjani K, Alemzadeh SA, Modarres M, Parvaresh MM, Hasehemi M, Naseripour M, Khanamiri HN, Askari S. Scleral buckling surgery for rhegmatogenous retinal detachment with subretinal proliferation. Eye (Lond). 2015;29:509–14.

12. Wong SC, Lee TC, Heier JS, Ho AC. Endoscopic vitrectomy. Curr Opin Ophthalmol. 2014;25:195–206.
13. Feltgen N, Heimann H, Hoerauf H, Walter P, Hilgers RD, Heussen N. SPR study investigators. Scleral buckling versus primary vitrectomy in rhegmatogenous retinal detachment study (SPR study): risk assessment of anatomical outcome. SPR study report no. 7. Acta Ophthalmol. 2013;91:282–7.
14. Feng H, Adelman RA. Cataract formation following vitreoretinal procedures. Clin Ophthalmol. 2014;8:1957–65.
15. Toyokawa N, Kimura H, Matsumura M, Kuroda S. Incidence of late-onset ocular hypertension following uncomplicated pars plana vitrectomy in pseudophakic eyes. Am J Ophthalmol. 2015;159:727–32.
16. Smith R. Suprachoroidal air injection for detached retina; preliminary report. Br J Ophthalmol. 1952;36:385–8.
17. Strampelli B. Use of gelatin sponge in the suprachoridal space in surgery of detached retina not reducible by immobilisation. Ann Ottalmol Clin Ocul. 1954;80:275–81.
18. Bauer F. The suprachorioideal fibrin implant as a new technic in surgery for retinal detachment. Klin Monatsbl Augenheilkd. 1966;149:76–9.
19. Hou J, Tao Y, Jiang Y, Wang K. In vivo and in vitro study of suprachoroidal fibrin glue. Jpn J Ophthalmol. 2009;53:640–7.
20. Sachsenweger R, Hartwig H. Suprachoroidal (subscleral) fillings of human fat for the operation of retinal ablations. Klin Monatsbl Augenheilkd. 1975;167:191–8.
21. Foulds WS, Aitken D, Lee WR. Experimental suprachoroidal plombage with a urethane based hydrophilic polymer. Br J Ophthalmol. 1988;72:278–83.
22. Poole TA, Sudarsky D. Suprachoroidal implantation for treatment of retinal detachment. Ophthalmology. 1986;93:1408–12.
23. Mittl RN, Tiwari R. Suprachoroidal injection of sodium hyaluronate as an 'internal' buckling procedure. Ophthalmic Res. 1987;19:255–60.
24. Szurman P, Januschowski K, Boden KT, Szurman GB. A modified scleral dissection technique with suprachoroidal drainage for canaloplasty. Graefe's Arch Clin Exp Ophthalmol. 2016;254:351–4.
25. Seuthe AM, Ivanescu C, Leers S, Boden K, Januschowski K, Szurman P. Modified canaloplasty with suprachoroidal drainage versus conventional canaloplasty—1-year results. Graefes Arch Clin Exp Ophthalmol. 2016;254:1591–7.
26. Seuthe AM, Szurman P, Januschowski K. Canaloplasty with suprachoroidal drainage in patients with pseudoexfoliation glaucoma – four years results. Curr Eye Res. 2020:1–7.
27. van Meurs JC, Van Den Biesen PR. Autologous retinal pigment epithelium and choroid translocation in patients with exudative age-related macular degeneration: short-term follow-up. Am J Ophthalmol. 2003;136:688–95.
28. Maaijwee K, Heimann H, Missotten T, Mulder P, Joussen A, van Meurs J. Retinal pigment epithelium and choroid translocation in patients with exudative age-related macular degeneration: long-term results. Graefes Arch Clin Exp Ophthalmol. 2007;245:1681–9.
29. Olsen TW, Feng X, Wabner K, Conston SR, Sierra DH, Folden DV, Smith ME, Cameron JD. Cannulation of the suprachoroidal space: a novel drug delivery methodology to the posterior segment. Am J Ophthalmol. 2006;142:777–87.
30. Szurman P, Boden KT, Januschowski K. Suprachoroidal hydrogel buckling as a surgical treatment of retinal detachment: biocompatibility and first experiences. Retina. 2016;36:1786–90.
31. El Rayes EN, Oshima Y. Suprachoroidal buckling for retinal detachment. Retina. 2013;33:1073–5.
32. El Rayes EN, Elborgy E. Suprachoroidal buckling: technique and indications. J Ophthalmic Vis Res. 2013;8:393–9.
33. El Rayes EN. Suprachoroidal buckling. In: Oh H, Oshima Y (eds): Microincision vitrectomy surgery. Emerging techniques and technology. Dev Ophthalmol (Basel, Karger). 2014;54:135–46.

34. El Rayes EN, Mikhail M, El Cheweiky H, Elsawah K, Maia A. Suprachoroidal buckling for the management of rhegmatogenous retinal detachments secondary to peripheral retinal breaks. Retina. 2017;37:622–9.
35. Mikhail M, El-Rayes EN, Kojima K, Ajlan R, Rezende F. Catheter-guided suprachoroidal buckling of rhegmatogenous retinal detachments secondary to peripheral retinal breaks. Graefes Arch Clin Exp Ophthalmol. 2017;255:17–23.
36. Mazinani B, Baumgarten S, Schiller P, Agostini H, Helbig H, Limburg E, Hellmich M, Walter P. Vitrectomy with or without encircling band for pseudophakic retinal detachment: a multi-centre, three-arm, randomised clinical trial. VIPER study report no. 1—design and enrolment. Br J Ophthalmol. 2016;100:405–10.
37. Heimann H, Hellmich M, Bornfeld N, Bartz-Schmidt KU, Hilgers HD, Foerster MH. Scleral buckling versus primary vitrectomy in rhegmatogenous retinal detachment (SPR study): design issues and implications. SPR study report no. 1. Graefes Arch Clin Exp Ophthalmol. 2001;239:567–74.
38. El Rayes EN. Supra choroidal buckling in managing myopic vitreoretinal interface disorders: 1-year data. Retina. 2014;34:129–35.
39. Yoon YH, Marmor MF. Rapid enhancement of retinal adhesion by laser photocoagulation. Ophthalmology. 1988;95:1385–8.
40. Hütz WW, Eckhardt HB, Kohnen T. Comparison of viscoelastic substances used in phaco-emulsification. J Cataract Refract Surg. 1996;22:955–9.
41. Antaki F, Dirani A, Ciongoli MR, Steel DHW, Rezende F. Hemorrhagic complications associated with suprachoroidal buckling. Int J Retina Vitreous. 2020;6:10.

Suprachoroidal Buckling for Myopic Macular Holes

Ehab N. EL Rayes and Mahmoud Leila

Introduction

Myopic macular hole (MMH) with or without retinal detachment is the extreme end of a spectrum of changes affecting people with pathologic axial myopia, known as myopic traction maculopathy (MTM). This term was coined by Panozzo et al. [1] using optical coherence tomography (OCT). It is a progressive pathology that starts with vitreomacular traction (VMT) and gradually progresses to the splitting of retinal layers leading to retinal thickening, macular retinoschisis, lamellar macular hole (LMH), full-thickness macular hole (FTMH), and eventually retinal detachment [2–5]. The pathogenetic cascade leading to MTM is multifaceted. It comprises of three forces targeting the retina and acting in opposite axis leading to its progressive splitting. This cascade is triggered by progressive enlargement of the posterior ocular wall, axial elongation and development of posterior staphyloma. The relatively inelastic retina fails to conform to the underlying choroid-sclera complex creating an inward traction towards the vitreous cavity, tangential traction at the vitreoretinal interface and an opposing traction force towards the outer global wall [1]. The rigidity of the retina is mainly attributed to the internal limiting membrane (ILM) and the retinal arterioles [1, 6].

Supplementary Information The online version of this chapter (https://doi.org/10.1007/978-3-030-76853-9_7) contains supplementary material, which is available to authorized users.

E. N. EL Rayes (✉) · M. Leila
Retina Department, Research Institute of Ophthalmology, Giza, Egypt

Surgical Management of MTM

In general, MTM is considered a stable condition that can remain stationary for years. Surgery is warranted only if the patient develops retinoschisis that encompasses the entire macula along with decreased vision, and in cases of foveal detachment, MMH, or MMH related retinal detachment (RD). Therefore, once MTM is diagnosed, monitoring of the patient is advised for timely intervention when required [3, 6].

The classic approach for treating macular holes using pars plana vitrectomy (PPV) combined with ILM peel does not fully address the pathogenesis of MTM related macular holes. The inward and tangential traction can be successfully eliminated by the posterior vitreous cortex and the rigid ILM removal. However, the outward traction caused by axial elongation and posterior staphyloma remains and may lead to recurrence even after initial successful MMH closure with vitrectomy and ILM peel. Hence, the management of MMH using this technique yielded variable success rates [7]. Closure rates of MMH ranged from as low as 33.3% reported by Matsumura et al. [8] and up to 90% and 91% according to Kwok et al. [9] and Wolfensberger et al. [10], respectively. Better results were achieved by using the inverted ILM flap technique [8, 11–13]. Some authors advocated refraining from ILM peel or resorting to a fovea-sparing ILM technique to avoid damaging the thin schitic macular area [2, 3, 14]. A more prudent approach would be the one that provided relief of both pathologic elements of bidirectional traction forces. This could be achieved by the addition of a macular buckle that flattened an existing posterior staphyloma, hence eliminating outward traction on the retina – choroid – sclera complex. Although macular buckle surgery has significantly improved the anatomical success rates of surgery for MMH and MMH retinal detachment [14–16], it remains a technically challenging procedure with a steep learning curve and set of complications that are related to the episcleral placement of macular explant over an extremely thinned posterior staphyloma. The reported complications included orbital fat prolapse during the procedure, inadvertent globe perforation, injury to vortex veins or ciliary vessels whilst placing sutures, torn sutures, submacular haemorrhage, indentation effect of the buckle leading to raised intraocular pressure (IOP), choroidal effusion due to mechanical compression on the choroidal circulation, buckle malposition, buckle extrusion, and localised retinal pigment epithelium (RPE) atrophy overlying the buckle [14–18].

Suprachoroidal Surgery for MTM

Successful surgery requires thorough knowledge of the anatomical features of the suprachoroid which is 10–34μm thick and is most compact posteriorly around the optic nerve, where the posterior ciliary arteries and nerves enter the eye, and around the vortex veins [1900] (see Chapter "Anatomy and Physiology of the Suprachoroidal

Space"). The rationale for the suprachoroidal approach to surgery in MTM is to circumvent the technical difficulty and potential complications of applying a scleral explant over the macula in highly myopic eyes. Suprachoroidal buckling underneath the macular area helps to counteract the anteroposterior traction. It can be performed solely if no RD is present or in combination with PPV in MMH associated with RD. In these cases, we did not attempt to peel the ILM to avoid the hazards of ILM peel in the presence of macular schisis [20–23]. The surgical procedure was chandelier-assisted. A conjunctival incision is made 4-mm behind the limbus at 12 o'clock position. A 3-mm circumferential sclerotomy is performed to expose the sclera and the suprachoroidal space. A bolus of viscoelastic is injected to protect the choroid for the atraumatic introduction of the catheter into the suprachoroidal space. Initially, we used a 450µm catheter prototype (Flextip Catheter; MedOne Surgical, Sarasota, Florida, USA). The catheter had the dual injection-illumination capability. One end was connected to a regular bright light source that illuminated a 39-gauge light fibre when placed in the suprachoroidal space. The other catheter end was connected to high-pressure tubing that delivered 20 mg/ml hyaluronic acid (HA) (Perlane; Q-med, Uppsala, Sweden). Perlane is a high-purity gel containing stabilised non-animal HA that creates a long-lasting three-dimensional gel network lasting 12–18 months with an excellent safety profile in dermal tissues. The catheter is fed through sclerotomy, sliding posteriorly against the scleral wall in the suprachoroidal space. A microscope mounted wide-field indirect viewing system is used to guide the catheter to the posterior staphyloma. At the edge of the staphyloma, a small amount of viscoelastic is injected to dissect and lift the choroid at the edge before pushing the catheter further into the posterior staphyloma. The illuminated tip of the catheter is visible underneath the choroid. Once the catheter is underneath the MMH, the viscoelastic is injected to create an indent and oppose the thin choroid to the retina creating a flat or a shallow convex configuration. The desired contour of the buckling effect is achieved under direct visualisation (Video 1). The newer Flex non-illuminated catheter (Flextip Catheter; MedOne Surgical, Sarasota, Florida, USA) offers the advantages of smaller diameter and obviating the need for a separate light port. The surgeon relies on direct visualisation of the indentation effect produced by the catheter to guide its path throughout the procedure (Fig. 1; Video 2). However, in the presence of high RD, it is difficult to detect the catheter and the illuminated catheter is used. Injection of viscoelastic is performed slowly to avoid causing an unwanted high buckle effect and consequent stretch of the short posterior ciliary arteries. At the end of the procedure, the circumferential sclerotomy is closed using 7/0 vicryl suture. In cases where the suprachoroidal buckle was combined with PPV, the indent stabilises the macula and facilitates the ILM peel, which can be a challenging manoeuvre in the presence of a detached schitic macula.

In a prospective noncomparative study, we reported 23 eyes of 23 patients with MTM including foveoschisis, LMH, MMH with posterior pole retinal detachment, and failed MMH repair after previous primary PPV with 12-month and 24-month follow up [22, 23]. All patients with myopic foveoschisis had resolution of schisis

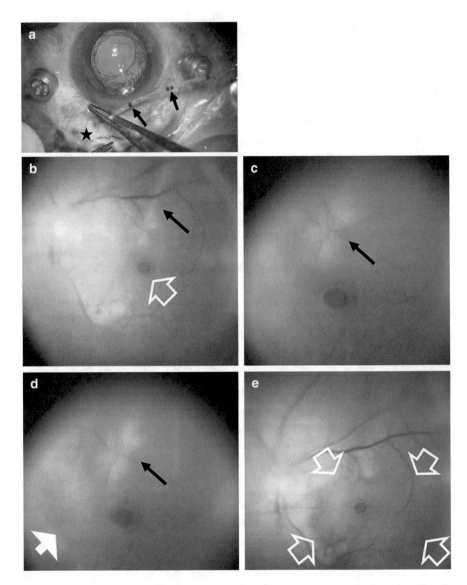

Fig. 1 Intraoperative snap shots show the suprachoroidal buckle procedure. (**a**) Insertion of modified El Rayes Flextip catheter into the suprachoroidal space through circumferential sclerotomy (asterisk). The new catheter has a non-illuminated tip and is graded by black markings placed 5-mm apart (black arrows) to gauge the distance travelled in the suprachoroidal space. (**b**) Surgeon's view of the fundus during guiding the catheter through the suprachoroidal space to the macular area. Note the indentation effect produced by the catheter (black arrow) superior to the macular hole (white arrow). (**c**) Initiation of injection of the viscoelastic (black arrow). (**d**) Note the change of the contour of the posterior pole as the viscoelastic continues to produce a buckle effect (white arrow). (**e**) Successfully completed procedure with full buckle effect underlying the macular area (white arrows)

over a period of 2–6 weeks. In patients with MMH and posterior pole RD, MMH closed successfully with the resolution of RD in 83% of eyes, the rest had persistent MH but resolved RD. Over 24-months of follow-up, we did not detect recurrence of foveoschisis or RD. It is noteworthy that after resorption of the viscoelastic and disappearance of the induced buckle effect, OCT scans showed that the choroid remained attached to the retina Fig. 2.

A complication experienced with surgery included choroidal track haemorrhage in 2 patients from trauma to thinned choroid at the edge of staphyloma, by threading catheter. Injection of a small bubble of viscoelastic upon reaching the edge of the staphyloma is therefore advised to gently displace the choroid for atraumatic passage of the catheter.

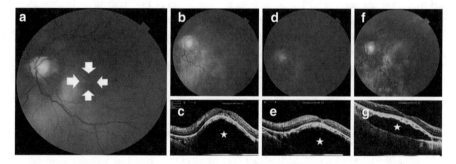

Fig. 2 Serial colour fundus photos and OCT images of the left eye of a patient with MMH and retinal detachment. (**a**) Pre-operative color fundus photo shows full-thickness macular hole (white arrows) with retinal detachment. The neurosensory detachment encompassed the entire posterior pole and extends beyond the arcades. Note the pale appearance of the retina and the lost choroidal pattern. (**b, c**) Colour fundus photo and OCT scan at one month follow-up visit after combined PPV and suprachoroidal buckle surgery. The retina is attached under silicone oil with successful MMH closure. OCT scan shows successful closure of MMH with dome-shaped elevation of the choroid and adherence to the overlying RPE. The suprachoroidal buckle effect appears as a hypo-reflective space beneath the choroid in the macular area (white asterisk). (**d, e**) Colour photo and OCT scan at 1-year follow-up visit. Note that the previously noted suprachoroidal buckle effect decreased in size due to gradual resorption of the viscoelastic (white asterisk). (**f, g**) Colour photo and OCT scan at 48-months visit. The silicone oil was removed and retina remains attached. OCT scan shows U-type closure of MMH with restoration of foveal microstructure. There was a reduction of the dome-shaped elevation produced by the suprachoroidal viscoelastic (white asterisk). The choroid remains adherent to the overlying RPE

Pearls and Pitfalls of Suprachoroidal Buckle Surgery

The technique of suprachoroidal buckle should not be attempted in the presence of over-thinned choroid (<100 μm) due to high risk of iatrogenic puncture of the choroid and insufficient choroidal tissue to produce the desired buckle effect.

The most significant complication during suprachoroidal buckle surgery is the development of haemorrhage due to trauma to the choroid. In order to minimise the incidence of bleeding from the choroid, the circumferential sclerotomy is best placed between 11–1 clock hours superiorly or between 5–7 clock hours inferiorly. The last scleral lamella should be opened using diathermy. The tip of the catheter should be pushed against the scleral wall as it is threaded into the suprachoroidal space. Proceed gently and stop at points of resistance and retry threading it again while injecting a small amount of viscoelastic. In patients with staphyloma, use viscoelastic to lift off the choroid before proceeding into the staphyloma. When deciding on the height of macular buckle aim to level the macula with the optic nerve or create a slight convex contour and avoid over-stretch of the suprachoroidal space and posterior ciliary arteries and nerves. During threading the catheter, track haemorrhage often develops along the trail of the catheter as it advances in the suprachoroidal space. This can be controlled by elevating the IOP.

Conclusion

The suprachoroidal buckle can be used to treat MTM – related pathology, performed either solely or in combination with PPV. The procedure requires thorough knowledge of the anatomical landmarks of the suprachoroidal space and the posterior pole, and surgical skills to execute it successfully.

References

1. Panozzo G, Mercanti A. Optical coherence tomography findings in myopic traction maculopathy. Arch Ophthalmol. 2004;122:1455–60.
2. Ruiz-Medrano J, Montero JA, Flores-Moreno I, Arias L, García-Layana A, Ruiz-Moreno JM. Myopic maculopathy: current status and proposal for a new classification and grading system (ATN). Prog Retin Eye Res. 2019;69:80–115.
3. Shimada N, Tanaka Y, Tokoro T, Ohno-Matsui K. Natural course of myopic traction maculopathy and factors associated with progression or resolution. Am J Ophthalmol. 2013;156:948–57.
4. Gaucher D, Haouchine B, Tadayoni R, Massin P, Erginay A, Benhamou N, et al. Long-term follow-up of high myopic foveoschisis: natural course and surgical outcome. Am J Ophthalmol. 2007;143:455–62.
5. Jo Y, Ikuno Y, Nishida K. Retinoschisis: a predictive factor in vitrectomy for macular holes without retinal detachment in highly myopic eyes. Br J Ophthalmol. 2012;96:197–200.
6. Ikuno Y, Gomi F, Tano Y. Potent retinal arteriolar traction as a possible cause of myopic foveoschisis. Am J Ophthalmol. 2005;139:462–7.

7. Ghoraba HH, Mansour HO, Elgouhary SM. Effect of 360° episcleral band as adjunctive to pars plana vitrectomy and silicone oil tamponade in the management of myopic macular hole retinal detachment. Retina. 2014;34:670–8.
8. Matsumura T, Takamura Y, Tomomatsu T, Arimura S, Gozawa M, Kobori A, Inatani M. Comparison of the inverted internal limiting membrane flap technique and the internal limiting membrane peeling for macular hole with retinal detachment. PLoS One. 2016;11(10):e0165068. https://doi.org/10.1371/journal.pone.0165068.
9. Kwok AKH, Lai TYY. Internal limiting membrane removal in macular hole surgery for severely myopic eyes. Br J Ophthalmol. 2003;87:885–9.
10. Wolfensberger TJ, Gonvers M. Long-term follow-up of retinal detachment due to macular hole in myopic eyes treated by temporary silicone oil tamponade and laser photocoagulation. Ophthalmology. 1999;106:1786–91.
11. Mete M, Alfano A, Guerriero M, Prigione G, Sartore M, Polito A, et al. Inverted internal limiting membrane flap technique versus complete internal limiting membrane removal in myopic macular hole surgery. A comparative study. Retina. 2017;37:1923–30.
12. Baba R, Wakabayashi Y, Umazume K, Ishikawa T, Yagi H, Muramatsu D, et al. Efficacy of the inverted internal limiting membrane flap technique with vitrectomy for retinal detachment associated with myopic macular holes. Retina. 2017;37:466–71.
13. Sasaki H, Shiono A, Kogo J, Yomoda R, Munemasa Y, Syoda M, et al. Inverted internal limiting membrane flap technique as a useful procedure for macular hole-associate retinal detachment in highly myopic eyes. Eye. 2017;31:545–50.
14. Mateo C, Burés-Jelstrup A, Navarro R, Corcóstegui B. Macular buckling for eyes with myopic foveoschisis secondary to posterior staphyloma. Retina. 2012;32:1121–8.
15. Ripandelli G, Coppé AM, Fedeli R, Parisi V, D'Amico DJ, Stirpe M. Evaluation of primary surgical procedures for retinal detachment with macular hole in highly myopic eyes. Ophthalmology. 2001;108:2258–65.
16. Ma J, Li H, Ding X, Tanumiharjo S, Lu L. Effectiveness of combined macular buckle under direct vision and vitrectomy with ILM peeling in refractory macular hole retinal detachment with extreme high axial myopia: a 24-month comparative study. Br J Ophthalmol. 2017;101:1386–94.
17. Ando F, Ohba N, Touura K, Hirose H. Anatomical and visual outcomes after episcleral macular buckling compared with those after pars plana vitrectomy for retinal detachment caused by macular hole in highly myopic eyes. Retina. 2007;27:37–44.
18. Siam AH, El Maamoun TA, Ali MH. Macular buckling for myopic macular hole retinal detachment. A new approach. Retina. 2012;32:748–53.
19. Bron AJ, Tripathi RC, Tripathi BJ. The choroid and uveal vessels. In: Wolff's anatomy of the eye and orbit. 8th ed. London: Chapman & Hall; 1997. p. 371–410.
20. El Rayes EN, Elborgy E. Suprachoroidal buckling: technique and indications. J Ophthalmic Vis Res. 2013;8(4):393–9.
21. El Rayes EN. Suprachoroidal buckling in managing myopic vitreoretinal interface disorders. 1-year data. Retina. 2014;34:129–35.
22. El Rayes EN. Suprachoroidal buckling. Dev Ophthalmol. 2014;54:135–46.
23. Mikhail M, El-Rayes EN, Kojima K, Ajlan R, Rezende F. Catheter-guided suprachoroidal buckling of rhegmatogenous retinal detachments secondary to peripheral retinal breaks. Graefes Arch Clin Exp Ophthalmol. 2017;255:17–23.

Suprachoroidal Drug Delivery

Shohista Saidkasimova

Introduction

Diseases of the posterior segment of the eye account for a significant proportion of visual impairment worldwide. Successful treatment results from both the most effective therapeutic agents and finding the best mode of delivery to achieve maximum bioavailability with minimal side effects whilst being comfortable for the patient.

Finding an optimal route for the drug delivery into the posterior segment of the eye is ongoing and presents challenges due to anatomical, physiological, and pharmacokinetic factors. Intravitreal, subretinal, subtenon, conjunctival, topical, oral and intravenous routes are all used to treat the posterior segment disease. Intravitreal injections have become the mainstem of the drug delivery for the posterior segment; however, their side effects are well documented [1, 2]. When choosing the optimal route for the delivery of drugs, it should aim to:

- Achieve lasting therapeutic levels in the target tissue
- Avoid penetration into undesirable structures (for example, anterior segment of the eye)
- Be safe and simple.

Use of suprachoroidal space (SCS) as the route of delivery of therapeutic agents has been explored since the 1970s [3–5]. An initial retrospective report of 10-year experience by Penkov et al. of 708 injections in 387 patients of a broad spectrum of drugs, including steroids for the treatment of chronic recurrent uveitis and diabetic macular oedema, antibiotics for the treatment of endophthalmitis and cytotoxic drugs after the excision of melanoma, suggested that it was safe and effective and was the delivery route of choice for patients with uveitis and diabetic retinopathy

S. Saidkasimova (✉)
Tennent Institute of Ophthalmology, Glasgow, UK
e-mail: shohista@doctors.org.uk

© The Author(s), under exclusive license to Springer Nature Switzerland AG 2021   117
S. Saidkasimova, T. H. Williamson (eds.), *Suprachoroidal Space Interventions*,
https://doi.org/10.1007/978-3-030-76853-9_8

[3]. A notable body of laboratory studies explored this route further (see Table 1). Suprachoroidal (SC) delivery allows a more targeted delivery into the posterior segment of the eye (retina and choroid in particular), compared with intravitreal and posterior subconjunctival (periocular) injection in animal models [7, 8]. Olsen et al. showed that the SC TA could remain for at least 120 days in the porcine choroid, retina and vitreous [9]. Use of SCS has the advantages of reduced exposure of drug into the vitreous cavity and anterior chamber, therefore reducing the secondary risks such as ocular hypertension and cataract. SC delivery also avoids entering the vitreous, considered an immune-privileged site with favourable conditions for bacterial survival and growth.

Fundamentals of Suprachoroidal Drug Delivery

Anatomical Considerations in the SC Drug Delivery

The suprachoroid is a potential space, and the structures within it are loosely adherent rather than firmly attached to each other. Little resistance is met when a substance is injected, but the amount of fluid that can be safely injected is limited by anatomical confinement and fluid dynamics. Evacuation of the fluid from SCS is dependent upon the difference between the intraocular, suprachoroidal and orbital pressures [10]. This difference of about 4 mm between the intraocular pressure (IOP) and suprachoroidal pressure ensures physiological apposition of suprachoroid and sclera. Such balance may be disturbed in cases of ocular hypotony, leading to transudation of fluid and opening of SCS. Injection of excessive amount of a substance into the SCS has the potential to disturb balanced hydrostatic pressure difference. Chen et al. have investigated different volumes of fluid injected into an animal model of rabbits and found that injection of up to 100µl volume was safe, but a higher amount was associated with a higher rate of complications, i.e. choroidal haemorrhage and ocular hypertension (OHT), backflow from injection entry, and serous sensory retina elevation from penetration through Bruch's membrane [11].

The distribution of a liquid substance was found to spread evenly in the SCS driven by gravitational forces [12]. An anatomical barrier that might impact the distribution of a substance was found in rabbit eyes along the long ciliary arteries [13]; however, this barrier does not exist in humans. A ring of numerous short ciliary nerves and arteries piercing the suprachoroid around the optic nerve pose more of a barrier to the distribution of drugs in the posterior pole of the eye in human suprachoroid making it more challenging to target the macula directly for treatment.

The outer blood-retinal barrier (BRB) consisting of retinal pigment epithelium (RPE) forms the main barrier to the drugs reaching the retina when delivered via suprachoroidal route. There is a strong relationship between the RPE permeability and molecular size. Bruch's membrane and choroidal tissue also prevent the passage of small molecules (up to 550 kDa). Animal studies have shown that the

Table 1 Preclinical studies on suprachoroidal deliveries

Year	Title	Model	Delivery instrument	Intervention	Control	Results
1998	Light microscopy of uveoscleral drainage routes after Gelatine Injections into the SCS [6]	Human eyes ex vivo (7)	23 g lacrimal cannula through a sclerotomy	Gelatine with Indian ink injection	None	Perivascular and perineuronal spaces of scleral vessels/nerves demonstrated; preformed channels in the anterior sclera drain directly into scleral veins
2002	Evaluation of a novel biomaterial in the SCS of the rabbit eye [4]	Rabbit in vivo	Olive tip cannula curved 600μm through sclerotomy	Injection of polymer (Polyorthoesther) to develop sustained release system	Hyaluronate	Polymer well tolerated, no inflammation on histology: Vacuoles formed with polymer, CR atrophy with hyaluronate
2006	Cannulation of the SCS: a novel drug delivery methodology to the posterior segment [9]	Macaca (1) in vivo, pig (94) in vivo, human eyes ex vivo	Flexible cannula (PDS; iScience interventional Inc.) through sclerotomy	In vivo cannulation technique through sclerotomy. SC fluorescein, ICG, TA injected	Fluorescein, ICG, TA injected	Complications of cannulation technique are described, incl ON damage and choroid injury with cannula. TA remained in the eye for 120 days. No changes on histology
2011	Pharmacokinetics of PP IVtI vs. microcannula SCI of bevacizumab in a porcine model [20]	Pig in vivo (62)	The cannula (PDS; iScience interventional Inc.) through sclerotomy	SC bevacizumab	IVt bevacizumab	IVt delivery of bevacizumab is longer sustained and better targeted for inner retina, no bevacizumab was detected after 7 days in SCI group, which offers better availability for RPE and photoreceptors. 7/30 eyes developed granulomatous reaction and vasculitis after IVtI bevacizumab

(continued)

Table 1 (continued)

Year	Title	Model	Delivery instrument	Intervention	Control	Results
2011	SC drug delivery to the back of the eye using hollow microneedles [24]	Rabbit, pig, human eyes ex vivo	Glass hollow microneedle different length (700, 800, 900, 1000μm)	Nanoparticles 20,100, 500, 1000 mcl delivery	Needle felt less resistance and travelled further with higher IOP	Smaller particles <100μm could enter SCS with shorter needles,800μm due to travelling between collagen fibres, larger particles needed a longer needle 1000μm and higher infusion pressure 250 kPa to enter SCS. SCI can be performed safely with hollow microneedle
2011	Effect and Distribution of Contrast Medium after Injection into the Anterior SCS in Ex Vivo Eyes [25]	Pig, dog eyes ex vivo	27 g cannula through sclerotomy	Latex injections and high frequency ultrasound (50 MHz) used to image the effect and distension of the SCS	None	SCS can expand in a dose-dependent manner, single anterior SCS injection can reach the ocular posterior segment
2012	Pharmacokinetic comparison of ketorolac after SC, IVt and intracameral administration in rabbits [26]	Rabbit in vivo (16)	32 g cannula via sclerotomy	SCI of ketorolac	Intracameral and IVt ketorolac	Liquid chromatography (HPLC) analysis. IVt ketorolac produced higher intraocular drug concentrations for a longer period compared with SC and i/cameral route. SCI reached effective drug level in the RC with short half-lives and low drug levels in the vitreous
2012	Comparison of SC drug delivery with subconj and IVt Routes Using Noninvasive Fluorophotometry [8]	Rats in vivo (10)	34 g needle	SC NaFl 100 mcg/ml	s/conj and IVt NaFl 100 mcg/ml	Na Fluoresceine fluorophotometry SCI achieved the highest concentration in choroid-retina

Year		Animal model	Needle	Formulation	Control	Results
2012	Targeted administration into the SCS using a microneedle [27]	Rabbit in vivo (6)	30 g hypodermic microneedle 700–800μm	SC Na Fluoresceine (NaFl) 600 mcg/ml, protein molecules 40 kDa & 250 kDa (=10 nm) dextran, 20 nm, 500 nm, 1 mcm & 10 mcm nanoparticles, bevacizumab (149 kDa)	IVt NaFl 6μg/ml	Fluorophotometry compared SC vs. IVt delivery, half-live for small particles in SCS was 1–8 h. Larger nanoparticles remained in SCS for months. No adverse effects reported
2013	Light-Activated, In Situ Forming Gel for Sustained SC Delivery of Bevacizumab [28]	Rabbit eyes ex-vivo; rats in vivo	30 g hollow microneedle	Light activated polycaprolactone dimethacrylate and hydroxyethyl methacrylate-based gel that sustains the release of stable, active bevacizumab	None	Bevacizumab release from 10-min, cross-linked gel was sustained for ~4 months
2013	Effect of choroidal perfusion on ocular distribution after IV or SCI in a perfused eye model [14]	Pig ex vivo (32)	27 g cannula	NaFl, carbocyanine dye and spectrophotometry in a perfused eye	NaFl, carbocyanine dye and spectrophotometry in non-perfused eye	Choroidal circulation reduces the tissue drug concentration of the hydrophilic drug suggesting an early clearance mechanism after SCS delivery. SCI allowed direct delivery to RC and limited exposure to the anterior segment

(continued)

Table 1 (continued)

Year	Title	Model	Delivery instrument	Intervention	Control	Results
2013	Treatment of acute posterior uveitis in a porcine model by SCI of TA using microneedles [29]	Uveitis in porcine model	33 g 850µm microneedle	0.2 mg and 2.0 mg of SCS TA	2.0 mg IVt TA injection	SC TA was as effective in reducing inflammation in a model of acute posterior segment inflammation. There were no adverse effects
2014	Particle-Stabilized Emulsion Droplets for Gravity-Mediated Targeting in the Posterior Segment [12]	Rabbit in vivo	30 g needle cannula 600–700µm	PEDs containing perfluorodecalin of 14µm, 25µm and 35µm diameter surrounded and stabilised by fluorescein-tagged, polystyrene nanoparticles	None	– Distribution of different molecular weight high-density PEDs with gravity should move PEDs toward the back of the eye, up to 50% of nanoparticles were in the most posterior quadrant near the macula immediately after injection and 5 days later – IOP elevation immediately after injection but dropped at 5 min and further at 20 min
2015	Formulation to target delivery to the ciliary body and choroid via the SCS of the eye using microneedles [30]	Rabbit in vivo	33 g needle cannula 750µm	Fluorescently tagged, polystyrene particles with various diameters (20 nm, 200 nm, 2µm, 10µm) suspended in HA or methylcellulose	Fluorescently tagged, polystyrene particles with various diameters (20 nm, 200 nm, 2µm, 10µm) were suspended in 50µL of BSS	Particles <10µm in BSS lead to spread of the particles over a portion of the SCS at the time of injection; additional spread occurs for up to 112 days after SCI. Particles in methylcellulose were immobilised at the site of SCI adjacent to the ciliary body for 60 days
2015	Real-Time Monitoring of SCS Following SCS Injection using OCT in Guinea Pig Eyes [31]	Guiney pigs in vivo	30 g needle	ICG or TA 50 mcg, 100, 150 mh	Duration of expansion of SCS is volume and formulation dependant	Expansion persisted for 24 h with TA, 180 min with ICG and 60 min with BSS; ICG had greater area of distribution than TA

Year	Title	Model	Needle	Formulation	Control	Results
2015	Safety and pharmacodynamics of SC TA as a controlled ocular drug release model [11]	Rabbit in vivo (12)	30 g needle	SC TA 50µL, 100µL, and 150µL	Subtenon TA 20 mg	SC TA group had less uveitis than subtenon group; SC complications: Choroidal haemorrhage, subretinal injection; volume was a significant contributor. Higher volume of SC TA increased risk of complications. Suspension increased risk of complications. 4 weeks after the IVI of proinflammatory LPS, uveitis was less significant in SC TA group
2016	Circumferential flow of particles in the SCS is impeded by the posterior ciliary arteries [13]	Rabbit in vivo/ human ex vivo	33 g hollow microneedle 750µm	50µL of 200 nm diameter red-fluorescent microspheres	None	The rabbit LPCA and the human SPCA were anatomical barriers to particle spread within the SCS
2017	Thickness and Closure Kinetics of the SCS Following Microneedle Injection of Liquid Formulations [32]	Rabbit in vivo/ex vivo	33 g hollow microneedle 750µm	25–150µL containing red-fluorescent particles, measured with US	25–150µL containing red-fluorescent particles, observed by FFI	With low-viscosity formulations, SCS expands to a thickness that remains roughly constant, independent of the volume of fluid injected. Increasing injection fluid viscosity significantly increased SCS thickness
2018	Targeted Drug Delivery in the Suprachoroidal Space by Swollen Hydrogel Pushing [33]	Rabbit in vivo/ex vivo	30 g hollow microneedle 750µm	1% HA with fluorescent polymer 2µm particles and a hydrogel formulation containing 4% HA; 9% NaCl	None	Drug particles can be targeted to the posterior SCS by HA hydrogel swelling and pushing: 76% of particles were delivered to the posterior SCS from SCI near the limbus

(continued)

Table 1 (continued)

Year	Title	Model	Delivery instrument	Intervention	Control	Results
2018	Ocular drug delivery targeted by iontophoresis in the suprachoroidal space using a microneedle [34]	Rabbit in vivo/ex vivo	30 g hollow microneedle 750μm	Iontophoresis at 0.14 mA for 3 min after injection of a 100μL suspension of nanoparticles	Injection of nanoparticles into the SCS of the rabbit eye ex vivo without iontophoresis	Iontophoresis using a novel microneedle-based device increased posterior targeting with >30% of nanoparticles reaching the most posterior region of SCS
2019	Collagenase injection into SCS to expand drug delivery coverage and increase posterior drug targeting [30]	Rabbit in vivo/ex vivo	30 g hollow microneedle 750μm	SCI of 1μm latex microparticles with collagenase	SCI of 1μm latex microparticles without collagenase	SCI of collagenase 0.5 mg/ml with incubation time of 4 h increased microparticle delivery coverage from 20% to 45% and enhanced posterior drug targeting
2020	Drug tissue distribution of tudca from a biodegradable SC implant vs. IV or systemic delivery [35]	Pig (46) in vivo	Implants placed via sclerotomy	Low- and high-dose SC, sustained-release with TUDCA	IV or IVt tauroursodeoxycholic acid (TUDCA, bile acid) delivery	The highest TUDCA tissue levels were obtained using IV delivery. Oral delivery was associated with reasonable tissue levels. Local delivery (IVtI and SCI) was able to achieve measurable local ocular tissue levels

Abbreviations: *IC* intracameral, *IV* intravenous, IVt intravitreal, *SC* suprachoroidal, *IVtI* intravitreal injections, *SCI* suprachoroidal injection. *SCS* suprachoroidal space, *PP* pars plana, *TA* triamcinolone acetonide, *OCT* optical coherence tomography, *RC* chorioretinal, *CR* chorioretinal, *PED* particle-stabilized emulsion droplets, *BSS* balanced salt solution, *LPS* lipopolysaccharide, *HA* hyaluronic acid, *LPCA* long posterior ciliary arteries, *SPCA* short posterior ciliary arteries, *US* ultrasound, *FFI* fundus fluorescence imaging outward permeability of drug (from the vitreous and retina to the choroid) exceeds the inward permeability (from SCS to the inner retina and vitreous) [14–16]. The retinal capillaries and the tight cellular monolayer of RPE cells only allow transport of small molecules <2 nm outward [17]. Amo et al. summarised the pharmacokinetics of retinal drug delivery and the relationship between the permeability and lipophilicity: the tight cellular monolayer of RPE cells has outward permeability of only 2×10^{-6} cm/s for hydrophilic molecules and eight times more for lipophilic molecules, whereas inward permeability is almost 100 times slower ($0.027 \times 10{-}6$ cm/s). However, this can also be advantageous for targeting the choroid as higher concentrations are achieved with suprachoroidal delivery compared with intravitreal delivery [8, 14, 18]. Of note, significantly higher levels of the drug in all ocular tissues were achieved with intravenous delivery compared with suprachoroidal or intravitreal delivery [19].

The choice of optimal route of drug administration is based on the target cells, their position in relation to BRB, the size of the molecule and its lipophilicity. An intravitreally administered drug bypasses the inner BRB of the retinal vasculature allowing a direct therapeutic effect on the retinal cells but has to travel through the RPE barrier to reach choroidal vasculature for therapeutic effect. In comparison, the suprachoroidal route has better availability for the choroidal vasculature, RPE and photoreceptor outer segments as shown on an animal model [20]. It avoids direct entry into the vitreous cavity, thereby theoretically decreasing the risks associated with intraocular delivery, i.e. endophthalmitis, retinal tears, cataract and ocular hypertension. Chen et al. found the level of the drugs in the retina after SCTA in a rabbit exceeded those in aqueous by 500 k times and those in vitreous by 200 times thereby reducing the potential ocular side effects associated with aqueous and vitreous exposure of the TA [11]. The blood flow in the choroidal vasculature is one of the highest in the human body and is 700 times higher than weight-adjusted blood flow in the liver [8]. Chen et al. found that the level of TA achieved in the retina after SC injection was 29 k times higher than after systemic administration, and the level in the anterior chamber was negligible at <1 ng/ml and very low in vitreous at 1912 ng/ml [11].

Histological Changes After the Injection

Einmahl et al. observed histologic changes at the site of injection of sodium hyaluronate into SCS with marked disorganisation of the architecture, pigmentation and vacuolisation of the outer retinal layers and focal loss of RPE with no inflammatory response in rabbit eyes [4]. These changes were less pronounced in eyes injected with more inert polyester polymer, where large vacuoles in SC melanocytes and thinning of overlying choroid developed [4]. Olsen did not find similar changes in a pig model [9]. In some clinical studies, no apparent lasting impact on SCS anatomy was noted at 1 month after SC TA injection [21, 22] but was reported in another study 3 months after injection [23].

Pharmacodynamics and Pharmacokinetics

Animal studies that investigated pharmacodynamics and pharmacokinetics of drugs in the suprachoroidal space are summarised in Table 1.

The choroid has a high blood flow, therefore the clearance from the suprachoroidal space is rapid and prevents sustainable levels reaching the neuroretina. This was demonstrated in an animal model comparing drug distribution in perfused with non-perfused eyes [14]. The distribution of balanced salt solution (BSS) within the SCS is very rapid: an injection of 0.2 ml of BSS leads to 1 mm opening of the SCS in height followed by rapid collapse within 10 s [12]. The distribution of the substance was influenced by molecular size and weight, and heavier molecules were found to travel further posteriorly [12]. Chen et al. (2015) reported a larger area of distribution of solution (indocyanine green, ICG) compared with suspension (TA). The volume injected also affected the distribution in the SCS, with the higher volume leading to broader distribution of the dye when different volumes of fluid were injected into the SCS of rabbit eyes [11].

Patel et al. used fluorophotometry to establish a correlation between the size of the molecules and their half-lives in the SCS of a rabbit eye [24]. Most macromolecules ranging in size from 40 kDa to 250 kDa (10mcm) dissolved from the SCS within 24 h. The half-life of a larger bevacizumab molecule was longer (~8 h) compared to smaller dextran molecule (~4 h). They also showed that the nano and microparticles, unlike the molecules, were not easily removed from the SCS and remained in a rabbit SCS for up to 2 months before animal sacrifice. Pre-equatorially injected particles were widely distributed in the SCS and choroid as far posteriorly as the optic nerve. Jung et al. successfully used collagenase to promote the wider distribution of a substance in the SCS and found that the incubation period of 4 h and the higher concentration of collagenase (0.5 mg/ml) was more effective in achieving that without significant impact on the structural integrity and scleral tensile strength in rabbit eyes [25].

The lipophilicity of the drug may act as a limitation to its wider spread. When comparing the transchoroidal migration of lipophilic drugs to hydrophilic drugs, Abarca et al. found that hydrophilic drugs were mainly eliminated by choroidal circulation whereas lipophilic drugs were not due to possible local binding with cell membranes of the choroid or Bruch's membrane [14]. Highly lipophilic TA suspension with low solubility and sustained release property has been the most explored therapeutic agent used in the SCS [11, 26–33]. SC injection of TA in a rabbit eye achieved max concentration in the sclera-choroid-retina lasting till day 29 before declining but was still detectable at day 91, whilst no TA was detected in the aqueous, and only traces were found in the vitreous [34].

The potential for the development of sustained drug delivery systems into the SCS has been explored by the use of biocompatible polymer [4, 35, 36], in situ cross-linked gel formation for sustained protein delivery [37], use of nanoparticles [36] and iontophoresis [38]. Another direction was to develop sustained release of anti-VEGF drugs in the SCS [37]. Injection of sustained-release suprachoroidal implants has been attempted in animals [19, 39], and the placement of fluocinolone acetonide intravitreal implant (Iluvien) into the SCS has been proposed in clinical practice [40].

Suprachoroidal drug delivery was compared with posterior subconjunctival and intravitreal routes using noninvasive fluorophotometry of sodium fluorescein in rat and rabbit animal models [8, 24] and achieved the highest retina-choroid concentration in the shortest time (25 times higher than intravitreal and 36 times higher than subconjunctival injection) and therefore was proposed as the most effective mode of delivery to the retina and choroid. Intravitreal injection had the longest half-life, most likely due to the time required to overcome BRB before reaching the rapid clearance by the choroidal vasculature [8]. Suprachoroidally injected sodium fluorescein cleared within 2 h, whereas intravitreal within 24 h, macromolecule of bevacizumab remained in the SCS longer before clearing by 24 h [7]. A similar comparison was made using the solution of ketorolac injected intracamerally, intravitreally and into SCS by Wang et al. but showed that intravitreal ketorolac achieved the higher drug concentrations and for a longer period (24 h) than suprachoroidal (8 h) and intracameral (4 h) injection [41]. This may be attributed to the different measurement technique or different biochemical properties.

Drug Delivery Technique

Delivery techniques into the SCS have been evolving [18, 42]. Initial deliveries employed full thickness scleral cutdown with cannulation of SCS [3, 43] (Fig. 1). Later the techniques have been refined on animal models with the use of small gauge (27, 32, 34 g) standard needles [8, 14, 41], however without the visual feedback and little resistance from the choroid the risk of choroidal injury and haemorrhage is high. An olive tip cannula was used to minimise such injury [4, 43]. Olsen et al. adapted the microcatheter used in glaucoma surgery for the Schlemm's canal in his animal study on porcine eyes [9]. Specially designed short hollow microneedles have been developed over the last decade to be long enough to penetrate sclera yet short enough to avoid injury to the choroidal vessels [36, 42, 44–47]. Patel et al. found that the SC injection was more successful in eyes with higher IOP, possibly due to less scleral surface deflection and deeper needle penetration and showed that the optimal size of needle for the injection is 1000 nm, although smaller particles can be delivered with shorter needles of 800μm by travelling between collagen fibres of inner sclera into the SCS [46]. Use of a microneedle allows a minimally invasive procedure that can be delivered in an office setting. Instruments designed for SC drug delivery include:

- SCS microinjector needle (Clearside Biomedical). The most commonly used, commercially available injectors in clinical trials are 900 and 1100μm microneedles [48] (Fig. 2).
- An olive tipped cannula (MedOne Surgical) 20, 23 or 25 g have been used for injecting high viscosity substance (Fig. 3).

Fig. 1 Insertion of blunt cannula though full thickness scleral incision

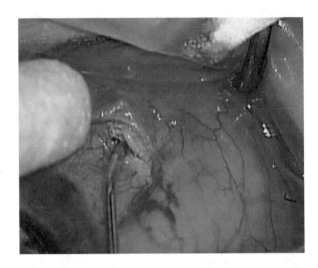

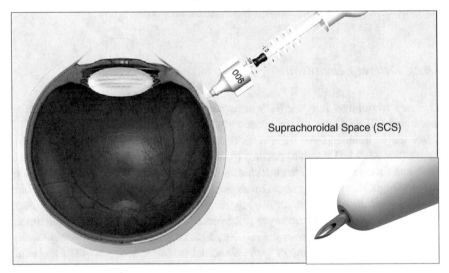

Fig. 2 Suprachoroidal microneedle (900μm) (Reproduced with permission from Clearside Biomedical)

- A suprachoroidal 450μm catheter for suprachoroidal injection (MedOne Surgical) can be connected to a regular bright illumination light source (see Chapter "Suprachoroidal Buckling for Myopic Macular Holes").
- Microcatheter (2004; iTRACK 400; iScience Interventional Corporation). The use of suprachoroidal catheters has been described in chapters "Suprachoroidal Buckling for Myopic Macular Holes" and "Suprachoroidal Delivery of Subretinal Gene and Cell Therapy".

Fig. 3 Olive tipped cannula, available in 20, 23 and 25 gauge (MedOne)

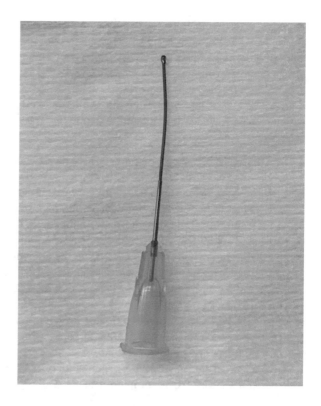

Scleral thickness is not uniform; it has been shown that superotemporal sclera is thinner than inferotemporal sclera by approximately 200μm [49, 50]. Axial length also correlates with scleral thickness, being thinner in high myopia and thicker in hypermetropia. This may influence the clinician's choice of the delivery technique.

Safety and Complications

Whilst the suprachoroidal injection (SCI) is a simple and quick procedure, a small number of complications documented in both preclinical and clinical studies included: backflow from the injection entry, needle injury causing choroidal haemorrhage, choroidal capillary bleeding (choroid haemorrhage away from needle entry), and serous sensory retina elevation from penetrating through Bruch's membrane [11, 28, 29]. Wang et al. reported extremely low plasma concentrations of ketorolac after suprachoroidal injection, suggesting that systemic absorption and therefore systemic side effects will be minimal [41]. Complications reported in the animal studies, i.e. endophthalmitis, choroidal tear, postoperative inflammation, scleral ectasia, wound abscess may have been exacerbated by the animal behaviour postoperatively [9]. Despite the initial concerns about the possible choroidal atrophy caused by SC injection in animal models, this was not confirmed in clinical studies: SC injection of CLS-TA may result in the expansion of the SCS but has not altered choroidal thickness [23]. Potential risk similar to the reported presumed air by vitrectomy embolisation syndrome (PAVE) [51] has not been reported with suprachoroidal drug delivery as yet.

Adverse events reported in the clinical trials were mild and moderate, and no serious adverse events were related to treatment. The most frequent complications included:

- Pain during injection was reported in 12% of patients at the time of injection and persisted 5% after the injection [26, 28].
- Ocular hypertension (OHT): a temporary rise in IOP is anticipated as it would with any additional volume introduced into a closed system, similar to intravitreal injections [52]. Pressure normalises after 5–20 min in an animal model [36]. Chen at al found that volume injected was a significant contributor to the OHT and that pressure rise was proportional to the amount of substance injected. IOP normalised within 20 min when $<$/$=$100mcl was injected, but a higher amount led to a more lasting OHT [11, 17]. Furthermore, a suspension (triamcinolone acetonide) had a higher rate of OHT than a solution (ICG) [11]. In a clinical setting, OHT was also observed [53]. However, in phase 3 clinical trial where only 100µl was used rate of post injection OHT was similar to the sham group [28].
- Choroidal haemorrhage was the most frequent complication in the human and in vivo animal studies involving cannulation of SCS [54] but was not reported in clinical trials with the use of microneedles [53].

Clinical Application

Targeted delivery of the drugs into the posterior segment without the side effects associated with anterior segment spread makes SCS an attractive route of delivery. Clinical administration of therapeutic substance into the SCS has been reported for uveitis, AMD, retinal vein occlusion (RVO), diabetic macular oedema (DMO) and choroidal melanoma [23, 26, 28, 33, 42, 55, 56]. Summary of the clinical trials is shown in Table 2.

Age Related Macular Degeneration (AMD)

A small retrospective case series of submacular SC injection of combined anti-VEGF (Bevacizumab) and Triamcinolone using a microcatheter in patients with advanced exudative AMD was reported as safe and beneficial for the reduction of retinal thickness and resolution of hard exudates [29].

Table 2 Clinical studies on suprachoroidal delivery

Study	Year	Phase	Title	Condition	No participants	Intervention	Control	Results	Complications
Retrospective [3]	1980	1	10 years' experience using the suprachoroidal method of administering drugs	Mixed	387	Mixed	None	SC delivery is safe and effective and is the delivery route of choice for patients with uveitis and diabetic retinopathy	Not available
Retrospective [29]	2012	1	Safety of submacular SC drug administration via a microcatheter	Exudative AMD	21	SC submacular bevacizumab and TA	None	Suprachoroidal infusion of drugs can be effective in reabsorbing massive hard exudates	1 cataract, 1 OHT
Retrospective [57]	2012	1	SC drug infusion for the treatment of severe subfoveal hard exudates	RVO, DMO	6	SC submacular bevacizumab and TA	None	Resolved hard exudates but no clinically significant improvement in vision, SC submacular TA is safe and effective	None
NCT01789320 [26]	2016	1/2	SC TA for noninfectious uveitis.	Uveitis	9	SC TA 4 mg	None	The safety and preliminary efficacy data support further investigations of SC TA for noninfectious uveitis.	ocular pain (4), OHT (0)

(continued)

Table 2 (continued)

Study	Year	Phase	Title	Condition	No participants	Intervention	Control	Results	Complications
SAPPHIRE [58]	2017	3	SC TA with IV Aflibercept in MO following RVO	RVO	480	SC TA + IV Eylea	IV Eylea	Terminated due to not achieving the primary 8 week efficacy endpoint with no additional benefit found for subjects receiving a corticosteroid in combination with an intravitreal anti-VEGF agent	Not available
TOPAZ [59]	2017	3	SC TA with IV anti-VEGF in MO following RVO	RVO	n/a	SC TA + IV Avastin or Lucentis	IV Avastin or Lucentis	Terminated early due to the early results obtained from the sister study, SAPPHIRE (CLS1003–301), which did not meet the 8 week primary efficacy endpoint	Not available
TANZANITE [33]	2017	2	SC TA for RVO	RVO	46	SC TA 4 mg and IV Eylea	IV Eylea	SC TA addition results in better VA, sustained reduction in CMO, and fewer injections	Cataract (1), OHT (4)
HULK [55]	2018	1/2	SC TA for DME	DMO	20	SC TA ± IV AntiVEGF		Improvement in DMO in all patients but treatment naive patients benefitted the most	inadvertent IVTA, OHT (2), cataract (3)
TYBBEE [53]	2019	2	SC TA with IV aflibercept vs. aflibercept alone in DMO	DMO	71	IV Eylea + SC TA	IVT Eylea	No difference in visual gain or SRT reduction but reduced frequency of injections	OHT (3) vs. 1 patient in control group

Study	Year	Phase	Title	Condition	N	Intervention	Comparator	Outcome	Safety
DOGWOOD [31]	2019	2	SC TA for MO due to noninfectious uveitis	CMO uveitis	22	SC TA 4 mg	TA	Safety analysis supported acceptable safety/ tolerability, significantly reduced central subfield thickness from baseline at 2 months, and significantly improved visual acuity	OHT (0)
PEACHTREE [28]	2020	3	Efficacy and safety of SC TA for MO due to noninfectious uveitis	CMO uveitis	160	SC TA 4 mg ± systemic steroids	Sham, ± systemic steroids	Significant gain in vision and reduction in central retinal thickness in patients with macular oedema secondary to uveitis treated with SC TA compared to sham group	OHT (0), cataract (0)
AZALEA [60]	2020	3	SC TA in noninfectious uveitis	Uveitis	38	SC TA 4 mg	TA	SCTA was safe and well tolerated. Efficacy parameters improved over 24 week period	OHT >30(2); cataract (1)
OASIS [61]	Ongoing	1/2	Safety and tolerability of SC AX following IV anti-VEGF in NV AMD	NV AMD	15	CLS-AX (tyrosine kinase inhibitor, axitinib) and Eylea		Ongoing	
NCT04417530 [62]	Ongoing	2	Safety and efficacy of SC AU-011 in small choroidal melanoma	Choroidal melanoma	31	Au-011	Sham	Ongoing	

Abbreviations: *IC* intracameral, *IV* intravitreal, *SC* suprachoroidal, *SCS* suprachoroidal space, *TA* triamcinilone acetonide, *RVO* retinal vein occlusion, *DMO* diabetic macular oedema

An alternative path for VEGF inhibition using Axitinib (tyrosine kinase inhibitor (TKI), Clearside Biomedical) with its broad VEGF blockade, currently approved for the treatment of renal cell carcinoma, is being investigated for the use in the SCS due to its potential prolonged effect for up to 6 months in the OASIS trial [61].

Rapidly developing direction of research as a potential treatment for the dry AMD is gene therapy, and suprachoroidal approach to gene vector delivery is being explored in animal and human eyes (ClinicalTrials.gov Identifier: NCT03846193) (see Chapter "Suprachoroidal Delivery of Subretinal Gene and Cell Therapy").

Retinal Vein Occlusion (RVO)

After an initial report of successful submacular suprachoroidal delivery of combined bevacizumab and Triamcinolone for the treatment of severe subfoveal hard exudates in a small prospective study of 6 patients [57], several studies explored its clinical benefits and risks.

Phase 2 randomised controlled trial (TANZANITE) evaluated suprachoroidal injection of triamcinolone acetonide as an aid to reduce the frequency of intravitreal aflibercept in patients with macular oedema secondary to RVO [23, 33]. The combination of SC TA with intravitreal Eylea was well tolerated and resulted in the reduced number of re-treatments in the combination arm compared with aflibercept alone, better visual gain and better sustained resolution of macular oedema.

Two Phase 3 sister trials on SC injection of TA with IVT antiVEGF for macular oedema secondary to RVO (Sapphire and TOPAZ) were initiated but were terminated due to failure to reach a primary 8-week efficacy endpoint and no identified additional benefit for subjects receiving a corticosteroid together with an intravitreal anti-VEGF agent [58, 59].

Uveitis

Uveitis has received targeted treatment via suprachoroidal route with the most benefit. The initial advantage of treating experimental uveitis with SC vs. intravitreal TA administration on an animal model was reported by Gilger et al. [30, 34]. Chen et al. confirmed the protective effect of suprachoroidal TA for the development of experimental uveitis induced by intravitreal injection of lipopolysaccharide in an animal model [11].

The clinical phase 2 DOGWOOD study was a small feasibility study which showed potential benefit of the SC TA [31] and paved the way for the PEACHTREE trial, which was the first completed Phase 3 clinical trial on suprachoroidal delivery recruiting 160 patients. It showed a significant gain in vision and reduction in central retinal thickness in patients with macular oedema secondary to noninfectious uveitis treated with SC TA compared to the sham group [28].

Diabetic Macular Oedema (DMO)

Rizzo et al. reported the potential benefit of SC delivery of combined SC TA and bevacizumab for severe exudative DMO [57].

The Hulk study was a prospective trial of suprachoroidal monotherapy with steroids [21, 55], enrolling 20 patients with treatment naive or previously treated DMO receiving either SC TA alone or in combination intravitreal antiVEGF repeated pro re nata. At 6 months, DMO improved in all patients, but treatment naïve group benefitted the most. No apparent lasting impact on SCS anatomy was reported [21]. The benefit of SC TA was also reported in cases of resistant DMO [63].

Phase 2 TYBBEE study looked at SC TA with IVT Aflibercept vs. Aflibercept alone in 71 DMO patients and did not show any visual benefit at week 24 but showed an almost two-fold reduction in the frequency of treatments [53]. No serious adverse events were observed, and ocular adverse events were low for both arms with a higher rate of elevated intraocular pressure in the SC TA group.

Melanoma

The anticancer properties of AU-011 (Belzupacap serotalocan), a novel bioconjugate capsid protein derived from the papillomavirus, were favourably evaluated on a rabbit model [64]. Its potential benefit in clinical practice using intravitreal approach has been proposed and studied [56, 65]. AU-011 (Aura Biosciences) is activated by 689-nm near infrared light (IR700DX) to induce acute necrosis of tumour cell. The drug selectivity binds to modified heparan sulphate proteoglycans (HSPGs) that are expressed on the tumour cell surface. Delivering AU-011 into the SCS can maximise bioavailability at the tumour site. A phase 2 randomised trial is currently underway to evaluate the safety and efficacy of AU-011, comparing SCI of AU-011 vs. sham in patients with primary indeterminate lesions and small choroidal melanoma (clinical trial NCT04417530) [66, 67].

Summary

Suprachoroidal delivery achieves high therapeutic levels of a drug in the choroid, RPE and the photoreceptor outer segments. This is short lived due to rapid clearance through high blood flow in the choroid and scleral permeability. Sustained release delivery systems may enhance the use of SC route and open possibilities for targeting pathology affecting the outer retina, choroidal vasculature and potentially sclera. The clinical trial results confirm that it may be the treatment delivery route of choice for posterior uveitis and may also reduce the burden of frequent treatments for

DMO. Conditions affecting the inner retina are limited by the outer BRB and therefore best targeted by the intravitreal approach.

Suprachoroidal delivery may have potential benefit in the early targeted treatment of choroidal neoplasm if cytotoxic drugs and viral-like particle bioconjugate (VPB) can be delivered at the primary site of tumour's growth.

References

1. Jager RD, Aiello LP, Patel SC, Cunningham ET. Risks of intravitreous injection: a comprehensive review. Retina. 2004;24(5):676–98.
2. Moshfeghi AA, Rosenfeld PJ, Flynn HW, Schwartz SG, Davis JL, Murray TG, et al. Endophthalmitis after intravitreal anti–vascular endothelial growth factor antagonists. Retina. 2011;31(4):662–8.
3. Penkov MA. ANM. A ten-year experience with the usage of the method of suprachoroidal administration of medicinal substances. Oftalmol Zh. 1980;35(5):281–5.
4. Einmahl S, Savoldelli M, D'Hermies F, Tabatabay C, Gurny R, Behar-Cohen F. Evaluation of a novel biomaterial in the suprachoroidal space of the rabbit eye. Investig Ophthalmol Vis Sci. 2002;43(5):1533–9.
5. Olsen TW, Aaberg SY, Geroski DH, Edelhauser HF. Human sclera: thickness and surface area. Am J Ophthalmol. 1998;125(2):237–41.
6. Krohn J, Bertelsen T. Light microscopy of uveoscleral drainage routes after gelatine injections into the suprachoroidal space. Acta Ophthalmol Scand. 1998;76(5):521–7. https://doi.org/10.1034/j.1600-0420.1998.760502.x.
7. Patel SR, Prausnitz MR. Targeted drug delivery within the eye through the suprachoroidal space. J Ocul Pharmacol Ther. 2016;32(10):640–1. https://doi.org/10.1089/jop.2016.0158.
8. Tyagi P, Kadam RS, Kompella UB. Comparison of suprachoroidal drug delivery with subconjunctival and intravitreal routes using noninvasive fluorophotometry. Li T, editor. PLoS One. 2012;7(10):e48188. https://doi.org/10.1371/journal.pone.0048188.
9. Olsen TW, Feng X, Wabner K, Conston SR, Sierra DH, Folden DV, et al. Cannulation of the suprachoroidal space: a novel drug delivery methodology to the posterior segment. Am J Ophthalmol. 2006;142(5):777–787.e2.
10. Emi K, Pederson JE, Toris CB. Hydrostatic pressure of the suprachoroidal space. Investig Ophthalmol Vis Sci. 1989;30(2):233–8.
11. Chen M, Li X, Liu J, Han Y, Cheng L. Safety and pharmacodynamics of suprachoroidal injection of triamcinolone acetonide as a controlled ocular drug release model. J Control Release. 2015;203:109–17.
12. Kim YC, Edelhauser HF, Prausnitz MR. Particle-stabilized emulsion droplets for gravity-mediated targeting in the posterior segment of the eye. Adv Healthc Mater. 2014;3(8):1272–82. https://doi.org/10.1002/adhm.201300696.
13. Chiang B, Kim YC, Edelhauser HF, Prausnitz MR. Circumferential flow of particles in the suprachoroidal space is impeded by the posterior ciliary arteries. Exp Eye Res. 2016;145(10):424–31.
14. Abarca EM, Salmon JH, Gilger BC. Effect of choroidal perfusion on ocular tissue distribution after intravitreal or suprachoroidal injection in an arterially perfused ex vivo pig eye model. J Ocul Pharmacol Ther. 2013;29(8):715–22. https://doi.org/10.1089/jop.2013.0063.
15. Tsuboi S, Fujimoto T, Uchihori Y, Emi K, Iizuka S, Kishida K, et al. Measurement of retinal permeability to sodium fluorescein in vitro. Invest Ophthalmol Vis Sci. 1984;25(10):1146–50.
16. Kimura M, Araie M, Koyano S. Movement of carboxyfluorescein across retinal pigment epithelium–choroid. Exp Eye Res. 1996;63(1):51–6.

17. del Amo EM, Rimpelä AK, Heikkinen E, Kari OK, Ramsay E, Lajunen T, et al. Pharmacokinetic aspects of retinal drug delivery. Prog Retin Eye Res. 2017;57:134–85.

18. Hartman RR, Kompella UB. Intravitreal, subretinal, and suprachoroidal injections: evolution of microneedles for drug delivery. J Ocul Pharmacol Ther. 2018;34(1–2):141–53.

19. Olsen TW, Dyer RB, Mano F, Boatright JH, Chrenek MA, Paley D, et al. Drug tissue distribution of tudca from a biodegradable suprachoroidal implant versus intravitreal or systemic delivery in the pig model. Transl Vis Sci Technol. 2020;9(6):11.

20. Olsen TW, Feng X, Wabner K, Csaky K, Pambuccian S, Cameron JD. Pharmacokinetics of pars plana intravitreal injections versus microcannula suprachoroidal injections of bevacizumab in a porcine model. Investig Opthalmol Vis Sci. 2011;52(7):4749. https://doi.org/10.1167/iovs.10-6291.

21. Lampen SIR, Khurana RN, Noronha G, Brown DM, Wykoff CC. Suprachoroidal space alterations following delivery of triamcinolone acetonide: post-hoc analysis of the phase 1/2 HULK study of patients with diabetic macular edema. Ophthalmic Surg Lasers Imaging Retina. 2018;49(9):692–7. https://doi.org/10.3928/23258160-20180831-07.

22. Huynh E, Chandrasekera E, Bukowska D, McLenachan S, Mackey DA, Chen FK. Past, present, and future concepts of the choroidal scleral interface morphology on optical coherence tomography. Asia-Pacific J Ophthalmol. 2017;6(1):94–103.

23. Willoughby AS, Vuong VS, Cunefare D, Farsiu S, Noronha G, Danis RP, et al. Choroidal changes after suprachoroidal injection of triamcinolone acetonide in eyes with macular edema secondary to retinal vein occlusion. Am J Ophthalmol. 2018;186:144–51. https://doi.org/10.1016/j.ajo.2017.11.020.

24. Patel SR, Berezovsky DE, McCarey BE, Zarnitsyn V, Edelhauser HF, Prausnitz MR. Targeted administration into the suprachoroidal space using a microneedle for drug delivery to the posterior segment of the eye. Invest Ophthalmol Vis Sci. 2012;53(8):4433–41.

25. Jung JH, Park S, Chae JJ, Prausnitz MR. Collagenase injection into the suprachoroidal space of the eye to expand drug delivery coverage and increase posterior drug targeting. Exp Eye Res. 2019;189:107824. https://doi.org/10.1016/j.exer.2019.107824.

26. Goldstein DA, Do D, Noronha G, Kissner JM, Srivastava SK, Nguyen QD. Suprachoroidal corticosteroid administration: a novel route for local treatment of noninfectious uveitis. Transl Vis Sci Technol. 2016;5(6):14. https://doi.org/10.1167/tvst.5.6.14.

27. Gu B, Liu J, Li X, Ma Q, Shen M, Cheng L. Real-time monitoring of suprachoroidal space (SCS) following scs injection using ultra-high resolution optical coherence tomography in guinea pig eyes. Investig Opthalmol Vis Sci. 2015;56(6):3623. https://doi.org/10.1167/iovs.15-16597.

28. Yeh S, Khurana RN, Shah M, Henry CR, Wang RC, Kissner JM, et al. Efficacy and safety of suprachoroidal CLS-TA for macular edema secondary to noninfectious uveitis. Ophthalmology. 2020;127(7):948–55.

29. Tetz M, Rizzo S, Augustin AJ. Safety of submacular suprachoroidal drug administration via a microcatheter: retrospective analysis of European treatment results. Ophthalmologica. 2012;227(4):183–9.

30. Gilger BC, Abarca EM, Salmon JH, Patel S. Treatment of acute posterior uveitis in a porcine model by injection of triamcinolone acetonide into the suprachoroidal space using microneedles. Investig Ophthalmol Vis Sci. 2013;54(4):2483–92.

31. Yeh S, Kurup SK, Wang RC, Foster CS, Noronha G, Nguyen QD, et al. Suprachoroidal injection of triamcinolone acetonide, CLS-TA, for macular edema due to noninfectious uveitis. Retina. 2019;39(10):1880–8.

32. Robinson MR, Lee SS, Kim H, Kim S, Lutz RJ, Galban C, et al. A rabbit model for assessing the ocular barriers to the transscleral delivery of triamcinolone acetonide. Exp Eye Res. 2006;82:479–87.

33. Campochiaro PA, Wykoff CC, Brown DM, Boyer DS, Barakat M, Taraborelli D, et al. Suprachoroidal triamcinolone acetonide for retinal vein occlusion: results of the Tanzanite study. Ophthalmol Retin. 2018;2(4):320–8.

34. Edelhauser HF, Verhoeven RS, Burke B, Struble BC, Patel SR. Intraocular distribution and targeting of triamcinolone acetonide suspension administered into the suprachoroidal space. Invest Ophthalmol Vis Sci. 2014:5259.
35. Jung JH, Desit P, Prausnitz MR. Targeted drug delivery in the suprachoroidal space by swollen hydrogel pushing. Investig Opthalmol Vis Sci. 2018;59(5):2069. https://doi.org/10.1167/iovs.17-23758.
36. Kim YC, Oh KH, Edelhauser HF, Prausnitz MR. Formulation to target delivery to the ciliary body and choroid via the suprachoroidal space of the eye using microneedles. Eur J Pharm Biopharm. 2015;95(1):398–406.
37. Tyagi P, Barros M, Stansbury JW, Kompella UB. Light-activated, in situ forming gel for sustained Suprachoroidal delivery of bevacizumab. Mol Pharm. 2013;10(8):2858–67.
38. Jung JH, Chiang B, Grossniklaus HE, Prausnitz MR. Ocular drug delivery targeted by iontophoresis in the suprachoroidal space using a microneedle. J Control Rel. 2018;277:14–22.
39. Barbosa Saliba J, Vieira L, Fernandes-Cunha GM, Rodrigues Da Silva G, Ligório Fialho S, Silva-Cunha A, et al. Anti-inflammatory effect of dexamethasone controlled released from anterior suprachoroidal polyurethane implants on endotoxin-induced uveitis in rats. Investig Opthalmol Vis Sci. 2016;57(4):1671. https://doi.org/10.1167/iovs.15-18127.
40. Al-Rayes E. Into the suprachoroidal space in the treatment of patients with DME, this location may offer an alternative for sustained-release corticosteroid implants. Retin Today. 2018:28–32.
41. Wang M, Liu W, Lu Q, Zeng H, Liu S, Yue Y, et al. Pharmacokinetic comparison of ketorolac after intracameral, intravitreal, and suprachoroidal administration in rabbits. Retina. 2012;32(10):2158–64.
42. Chiang B, Jung JH, Prausnitz MR. The suprachoroidal space as a route of administration to the posterior segment of the eye. Adv Drug Deliv Rev. 2018;126:58–66.
43. Poole TA, Sudarsky RD. Suprachoroidal implantation for the treatment of retinal detachment. Ophthalmology. 1986;93(11):1408–12.
44. Rai UDJP, Young SA, Thrimawithana TR, Abdelkader H, Alani AWG, Pierscionek B, et al. The suprachoroidal pathway: a new drug delivery route to the back of the eye. Drug Discov Today. 2015;20(4):491–5.
45. Jung JH, Chiang B, Grossniklaus HE, Prausnitz MR. Suprachoroidal space using a microneedle. 2019;14–22.
46. Patel SR, Lin ASP, Edelhauser HF, Prausnitz MR. Suprachoroidal drug delivery to the back of the eye using hollow microneedles. Pharm Res. 2011;28(1):166–76.
47. Chitnis GD, Verma MKS, Lamazouade J, Gonzalez-Andrades M, Yang K, Dergham A, et al. A resistance-sensing mechanical injector for the precise delivery of liquids to target tissue. Nat Biomed Eng. 2019;3(8):621–31.
48. Barakat M, Cherry Wan BK. Post hoc analysis of clinical suprachoroidal injection experience across indications. Invest Ophthalmol Vis Sci. 2020;61(e7):4954.
49. Vurgese S, Panda-Jonas S, Jonas JB. Scleral thickness in human eyes. Vavvas D, editor. Vavvas D. PLoS One. 2012;7(1):e29692. https://doi.org/10.1371/journal.pone.0029692.
50. Wan C, Kapik B, Wykoff CC, Henry CR, Barakat MR, Shah M, et al. Clinical characterisation of suprachoroidal injection procedure utilising a microinjector across three retinal disorders. Transl Vis Sci Technol. 2020;9(11):27.
51. Morris R, Sapp MR, Oltmanns MH, Kuhn F. Presumed air by vitrectomy embolisation (PAVE): a potentialy fatal syndrome. Br J Ophthmol. 2014;98(6);765–8. Epub 2013 Jun 21. PMID:23793850. PMCID: PMC4033178. https://doi.org/10.1136/bjophthalmol-2013-303367.
52. Benz MS, Albini TA, Holz ER, Lakhanpal RR, Westfall AC, Iyer MN, et al. Short-term course of intraocular pressure after intravitreal injection of triamcinolone acetonide. Ophthalmology. 2006;113(7):1174–8.
53. Barakat MR, Wykoff CC, Gonzalez V, Hu A, Marcus D, Zavaleta E, et al. Suprachoroidal CLS-TA plus intravitreal aflibercept for diabetic macular edema: a randomised, double-masked,

parallel-design, controlled study. Ophthalmol Retin. 2020:1–11. https://doi.org/10.1016/j.oret.2020.08.007.

54. Antaki F, Dirani A, Ciongoli MR, Steel DHW, Rezende F. Hemorrhagic complications associated with suprachoroidal buckling. Int J Retin Vitr. 2020:1–12. https://doi.org/10.1186/s40942-020-00211-6.

55. Wykoff CC, Khurana RN, Lampen SIR, Noronha G, Brown DM, Ou WC, et al. Suprachoroidal triamcinolone acetonide for diabetic macular edema. Ophthalmol Retin. 2018;2(8):874–7.

56. Mruthyunjaya P, Schefler AC, Kim IK, Bergstrom C, Demirci H, Tsai T, et al. A phase 1b/2 open-label clinical trial to evaluate the safety and efficacy of AU-011 for the treatment of choroidal melanoma. Invest Ophthalmol Vis Sci. 2020;61(7):4025.

57. Rizzo S, Ebert FG, Di Bartolo E, Barca F, Cresti F, Augustin C, et al. Suprachoroidal drug infusion for the treatment of severe subfoveal hard exudates. Retina. 2012;32(4):776–84.

58. Suprachoroidal injection of triamcinolone acetonide with IVT aflibercept in subjects with macular edema following RVO (SAPPHIRE). ClinicalTrials.gov Identifier NCT02980874. 2018.

59. Suprachoroidal injection of triamcinolone acetonide with IVT anti-VEGF in subjects with macular Edema following RVO (TOPAZ). ClinicalTrials.gov Identifier NCT03203447. 2018. https://clinicaltrials.gov/ct2/show/NCT03203447?term=suprachoroidal+topaz&draw=2&rank=1

60. Suprachoroidal injection of CLS-TA in subjects non-infectious uveitis (AZALEA). Clin Identifier NCT03097315. https://clinicaltrials.gov/ct2/show/NCT03097315?term=Azalea&draw=2&rank=1

61. Safety and tolerability study of suprachoroidal injection of CLS-AX following anti-VEGF therapy in neovascular AMD (OASIS). Clin Identifier. 2020;NCT0462612. https://clinicaltrials.gov/ct2/show/NCT04626128?term=OASIS+suprachoroidal&draw=2&rank=1

62. Phase 2 trial to evaluate safety and efficacy of AU-011 via suprachoroidal administration in subjects with primary indeterminate lesions and small choroidal melanoma. Clin Identifier NCT04417530. https://clinicaltrials.gov/ct2/show/NCT04417530

63. Tayyab H, Ahmed CN, Sadiq MAA. Efficacy and safety of suprachoroidal triamcinolone acetonide in cases of resistant diabetic macular edema. Pakistan J Med Sci. 2020;36(2):42–7.

64. Kines RC, Varsavsky I, Choudhary S, Bhattacharya D, Spring S, McLaughlin R, et al. An infrared dye–conjugated virus-like particle for the treatment of primary uveal melanoma. Mol Cancer Ther. 2018;17(2):565–74. https://doi.org/10.1158/1535-7163.MCT-17-0953.

65. Shields CL, Lim L-AS, Dalvin LA, Shields JA. Small choroidal melanoma. Curr Opin Ophthalmol. 2019;30(3):206–14.

66. Phase 2 trial to evaluate safety and efficacy of AU-011 via suprachoroidal administration in subjects with primary indeterminate lesions and small choroidal melanoma. https://clinicaltrials.gov/ct2/show/NCT04417530

67. Savinainen A, Grossniklaus H, Kang S, Rasmussen C, Bentley E, Krakova Y, et al. Ocular distribution and efficacy after suprachoroidal injection of AU-011 for treatment of ocular melanoma. Invest Ophthalmol. 2020;61(7):3615.

Suprachoroidal Delivery of Subretinal Gene and Cell Therapy

David Xu, M. Ali Khan, and Allen C. Ho

Introduction

Clinical trial investigation of gene- and stem cell-based therapies has greatly expanded in recent years with treatment aimed at a diverse array of inherited retinal disorders (IRDs) [1, 2] and non-hereditary retinal degenerations [3]. Conditions that have been evaluated include *RPE65*-associated Leber's congenital amaurosis (LCA), retinitis pigmentosa (RP), Stargardt disease, and age-related macular degeneration (AMD), amongst others. The 2017 approval of voretigene neparvovec-rzyl (Luxturna, Spark Therapeutics, Philadelphia, PA, USA) by the U.S. Food and Drug Administration to treat biallelic *RPE65* mutation-associated retinal dystrophy, the first approved gene therapy, was the fruition of decades of genetic research and marked the dawn of the gene therapy era for ocular conditions and medicine in general.

Access to the subretinal and/or suprachoroidal space (SCS) is of particular interest for targeted delivery of retinal genetic or cellular therapeutics. For most retinal diseases, the target cell layer is usually the retinal photoreceptors or the retinal pigment epithelium (RPE) which are in or adjacent to the outer retina [4], although some inner retinal conditions affecting Muller cells [5] or ganglion cells [6] have been studied.

Gene and cell delivery methods need to transfer a sufficiently high concentration of the therapeutic agent to the target tissue, which is challenging due to the contiguous, multi-layered arrangement of the retina and RPE. Internally, the retina is bounded by the relatively impermeable internal limiting membrane (ILM) which can bind and prevent diffusion of viral vectors from the vitreous into the retina [7].

D. Xu · M. A. Khan · A. C. Ho (✉)
Retina Service, Wills Eye Hospital, Thomas Jefferson University Hospitals, Philadelphia, PA, USA
e-mail: makhan@midatlanticretina.com; acho@midatlanticretina.com

© The Author(s), under exclusive license to Springer Nature Switzerland AG 2021
S. Saidkasimova, T. H. Williamson (eds.), *Suprachoroidal Space Interventions*,
https://doi.org/10.1007/978-3-030-76853-9_9

Externally, the retina is bounded by the RPE which has intercellular tight junctions that comprise a crucial part of the blood-retina barrier. As successful therapy depends on close spatial approximation to the target tissue, several surgical approaches for targeted delivery of novel gene- and cell-based therapies have been developed. The subject of this chapter is to review the role of the suprachoroidal space (SCS) as a route of administration for gene and cell therapy treatment modalities.

Current Landscape of Retinal Therapies

Gene Versus Cell Therapy

It is important first to discuss the overarching goal and biomolecular methods to achieve gene and cell therapy for eye diseases. Gene therapy seeks to augment, suppress, or edit a gene of interest, or introduce one or more new genes to produce a desirable effect [3, 8].Targetcells maybe those with a genetic defect, as in IRDs, or a neighbouring cell type that can be utilised to produce a desired therapeutic protein–in other words, to create a protein "biofactory."

On the other hand, cell therapy involves the delivery of whole cells to support, repair, or replace damaged cells [9, 10]. Replacement of damaged cells may be termed "regenerative" cell therapy, while support or repair of existing, injured cells may be termed "trophic" cell therapy. In both cases, the goal of cell therapy is to restore native function.

Gene Therapy

The advantage of gene therapy over traditional pharmacological approaches is that it can directly address a specific genetic defect rather than its downstream cellular effects. Also, it offers the potential for durable treatment response from a single treatment when used to create an ocular protein biofactory. Different gene therapy strategies have been developed, which can be categorised as gene augmentation, gene-specific targeting, and genome editing [3]. Gene augmentation has been most extensively studied for IRDs and seeks to introduce a functional copy of a gene to replace a missing or faulty host gene. Delivery strategies involve the selection of a delivery vehicle (most commonly a viral vector) and a method of administration to target cells. For example, gene augmentation was first successfully utilised to treat type 2 LCA due to defective*RPE65* [11–13]. The gene encodes all-trans retinyl ester isomerase, and patients with biallelic mutations of the gene develop severe infantile-onset vision loss. Patients given a subretinal injection of a recombinant adeno-associated virus (AAV2)vector carrying a normal copy of *RPE65*DNA demonstrated improved visual acuity, navigational abilities, and functional visual gains [12].A number of other IRDs have been evaluated using AAV-based vector-transgene products. Phase 1/2 clinical trials for choroideremia were conducted to replace the mutated *CHM* gene using an AAV2 vector [14–16]. Gene augmentation has also entered clinical testing for Leber's hereditary optic neuropathy [6, 17, 18], retinitis pigmentosa [19], achromatopsia [20, 21], X-linked retinoschisis [5] and others. Most ocular gene therapy trials have used AAV-based viral vectors [22, 23], although a few have used lentiviral vectors, for example, in *ABCA4*-associated Stargardt's disease [24–27]. A major limitation of AAV vectors is their payload limit of approximately 4.8 kilobases (kb). In contrast, lentiviruses can package a gene product up to 9–10 kb long [28].

Gene delivery has also been studied for non-hereditary retinal degenerations such as neovascular AMD [29–31]and non-neovascular AMD [32]. Most clinical trials have focused on introducing a new gene which encodes for a protein with potential desirable effects, rather than replacing a faulty gene. Current therapies are centred around vascular endothelial growth factor (VEGF) suppression. The benefit of intravitreal anti-VEGF therapy for neovascular AMD has been demonstrated with monoclonal antibodies, such as ranibizumab, and soluble decoy receptors, such as aflibercept [33–35]. While they are an effective treatment modality, frequent re-injection is required to maintain their effect. Gene delivery trials have been conducted to allow transduced retinal cells to natively express anti-VEGF proteins, including soluble FMS-like tyrosine kinase-1 (s-Flt-1), endostatin/angiostatin,andranibizumab [29–31]. For non-neovascular AMD, clinical trials are exploring AAV-based therapy to produce complement regulatory protein sCD59 (Hemera Biosciences, Waltham, MA, USA) [32] and complement factor I (Gyroscope Therapeutics, London, United Kingdom) [36].

Cell Therapy

A large array of cell types and cellular replacement strategies have been under investigation for retinal degenerations and IRDs [9, 10]. The transient dosing strategy uses multipotent stem cells or progenitor cells to secrete neuroprotective, trophic or immune-modulatory factors to the target tissue. The permanent implantation strategy uses stem cell-derived photoreceptor or RPE cells to replace damaged or atrophied host cells. Human embryonic stem cells (hESCs) [37–40], induced pluripotent stem cells (iPSCs) [41], and human umbilical tissue-derived cells (hUTCs) [42, 43] are among many cell lines which have undergone preclinical and clinical investigation.

A phase 1/2a trial of ahESC-derived RPE monolayer seeded on a synthetic substrate (California Project to Cure Blindness-RPE1, California, USA) was conducted in patients with advanced non-neovascular AMD [38–40]. Subretinal implantation of the cell layer using a custom insertion forceps was well tolerated, and the graft could be reliably positioned within areas of geographic atrophy (GA). Another phase 1 trial of a hESC-RPE patch on a synthetic basement membrane was performed in patients with neovascular AMD [37]. The procedure led to significant vision gains although only 2 patients were entered in the study. Palucorcel, or CNTO-2476 (Janssen Research and Development, Beerse, Belgium), is a cryopreserved formulation of hUTCs. Subretinal delivery of the cell suspension adjacent to areas of GA in non-neovascular AMD met safety and tolerability endpoints in a phase 1/2 clinical trial [42, 43].

Approaches for Retinal Therapy

The anatomy of the eye and ocular coats provides several benefits for gene or cellular delivery. First, the eye is small and requires a relatively low quantity of the therapeutic agent. Second, the blood-retina barrier at the RPE creates an immune-privileged space which limits host inflammatory response. Third, the confined anatomy of the eye limits systemic exposure. Finally, the posterior segment can be assessed using a variety of imaging modalities to measure treatment response. These traits make the eye an attractive candidate organ for evaluating novel therapies.

Different approaches have been used for delivering therapeutics to the retina. These include intravitreal injection (IVI), subretinal injection via pars plana vitrectomy (PPV), suprachoroidal injection, and subretinal injection via a suprachoroidal-tunnelledmicrocatheter [44].Access via the suprachoroidal space (SCS) has certain advantages and disadvantages, but should first be contrasted to the other approaches.

Intravitreal Delivery

IVI has been evaluated for retinal gene therapy. The treatment can be performed in the office with topical anaesthesia and incurs a low risk of procedure-related complications. The method has been applied for the treatment of X-linked retinoschisis [5], Leber's hereditary optic neuropathy [17, 18, 45–47], and experimental models of glaucoma [6]. Historically, the technique has shown limited clinical success, thought to be secondary to poor penetration of viral vectors through the internal limiting membrane, and transduction is often limited to the inner retinal layers [7]. Another disadvantage is that the intravitreal delivery of viral vector proteins may trigger a host immune response. Exposure to pre-existing neutralising antibodies (NAbs) in the vitreous can stimulate inflammation and reduce vector integrity and yield [48–50]. Current IVI-based gene therapy clinical trials for neovascular AMD are employing new, modified viral vectors such as AAV.7 m8 (Adverum Biotechnologies, Menlo Park, California, USA) which may have increased affinity for retinal target tissue [51].

Subretinal Delivery

The majority of retinal gene and cellular therapies have been surgically delivered to the subretinal space. This method involves PPV in the operating room, induction of a posterior vitreous detachment, and creation of a retinotomy—an opening through the ILM and retina—to gain access to the subretinal space [44, 52]. The viral solution is injected into the potential space between the photoreceptor layer and the RPE forming a localised retinal detachment, or "bleb," where viral particles diffuse. Subretinal injection of AAV vectors can lead to strong and long-lasting transgene expression in the photoreceptors and RPE [53, 54]. Due to the relative immune-privileged nature of the subretinal space, viruses are not exposed to NAbs, and if needed, subsequent dosages can be delivered without clinically observed immune response [55]. PPV is associated with procedure-related complications including cataract progression and the rare risk of retinal detachment. Subretinal delivery also induces transient detachment of the retina, which can injure photoreceptors, and detachment of the fovea can lead to persistently decreased visual acuity or precipitate macular hole formation [53]. Furthermore, the trajectory of subretinal fluid migration may be unpredictable during bleb creation, and the size and location of the bleb may be important for therapeutic effect. Because transduction occurs only in tissue exposed to the virus-containing fluid, multiple retinotomies may be required to treat the desired area. Finally, reflux of cellular material into the vitreous through the retinotomy can reduce transduction efficiency and potentially lead to epiretinal membrane formation over the macula [56].

Suprachoroidal Delivery

The potential disadvantages of the transvitreal approach have in part stimulated the design and testing of suprachoroidal delivery. Suprachoroidal drug delivery has been extensively evaluated for a number of small molecules [57–61], corticosteroids [62–64], and monoclonal antibodies [65]. Injection into the SCS can be performed with a standard needle, transscleral microneedle or cannulation with a flexible microcatheter. To date, the best studied suprachoroidal therapy is the injection of corticosteroid using a transscleral microneedle for the treatment of macular oedema secondary to noninfectious uveitis and retinal vein occlusion [62–64]. In the context of retinal gene and cellular therapy, the SCS is attractive as a route to access the subretinal space because it allows for treatment of the retina and RPE without the procedure-associated risks of PPV, retinotomy creation, and the immunogenicity of intravitreal injection. Suprachoroidal gene delivery potentially allows for widespread retinal/RPE transduction, and, if further refined, may allow gene therapy to be completed as an office-based procedure rather than in the operating room.

Subretinal cell delivery via the SCS has successfully been applied in human trials [42, 66]. Genetic or cellular therapy can be delivered into the subretinal space using a needle or suprachoroidal tunnelled microcatheter that is advanced toward the posterior pole [42, 66, 67]. Although suprachoroidal delivery avoids the need for vitrectomy and retinotomy creation, potential procedure-related complications still exist including suprachoroidal haemorrhage and retinal perforation.

Methods to Access the Suprachoroidal Space

Standard Hypodermic Needle

The simplest method for suprachoroidal injection is using a standard hypodermic needle. The needle is advanced through the sclera adjacent to the limbus in a tangential angle until the tip enters the SCS [67]. When the surgeon feels a decrease in resistance, fluid is slowly injected, which expands the suprachoroidal potential space. Small molecules injected near the limbus diffuse circumferentially around the eye, allowing for treatment of a large portion of the retina [57]. The potential for gene therapy via direct suprachoroidal injection was tested using RGX-314 (REGENXBIO, Rockville, Maryland, USA), a recombinant AAV8 vector expressing anti-VEGF Fab, in non-human primate and pig eyes [67]. A single suprachoroidal injection led to widespread retinal transduction and suppression of VEGF-induced vascular leakage. The drawbacks of the freehand technique include a procedure learning curve and possibility that the needle could be advanced too far, leading to inadvertent subretinal or intravitreal injection.

Transscleral Microneedle

Suprachoroidal gene delivery using a specialised, transscleral, limited depth microneedle has been evaluated in animal models [68]. In contrast to a standard, long hypodermic needle, the length of a suprachoroidal microneedle is typically only 700–1100 microns which limits over-penetration and allows for reproducible access to the SCS [69]. Microneedle injection can be performed in the office setting with local anaesthesia similar to intravitreal injection, although the location of injection is typically farther posterior in the mid-quadrant of the globe. Suprachoroidal administration of an AAV8 vector expressing green fluorescent protein (GFP) in rhesus macaques demonstrated widespread, peripheral retinal transduction at 1 month [68]. There are limitations with the delivery of viral products in the SCS. In the same study, GFP expression after 2–3 months was no longer present, and suprachoroidal administration was associated with significant localised infiltration of inflammatory cells in the retina and choroid. Retinal transduction from the suprachoroidal approach may be less efficient than subretinal administration due to rapid blood flow and clearance of viral particles from the choriocapillaris [70].

Tunnelled Microcatheter

To direct treatment toward the posterior pole, another method of suprachoroidal delivery has been evaluated using a tunnelled microcatheter passed through the suprachoroidal space (Fig. 1) [71]. This surgical method was initially explored using a 250 microns-diameter microcatheter, the iTrack 250A (iScience Interventional Corporation, Menlo Park, California, USA). This flexible catheter was originally designed for cannulation of Schlemm's canal and had an illuminated light at the cannula tip for localisation. A limbal conjunctival peritomy is first created, and a radial scleral cut down is made 3–4 mm posterior to the limbus to expose the choroid. The catheter is then introduced into the SCS where it travels between the choroid and scleral wall and is advanced posteriorly toward the optic nerve. The path of the catheter tip can be visualised using indirect ophthalmoscopy to guide it into its final position. This method was used for successful transduction of the retina by an AAV8 vector in rabbits [72].

The subretinal injection can also be performed through a suprachoroidal approach [42, 43, 66]. The first trans choroidal, subretinal delivery method utilised a similar tunnelled, illuminated microcatheter (iTrack 275, iScience Interventional Corporation, Menlo Park, California, USA) to deliver subretinal Palucorcel,or CNTO-2476,composed of human umbilical tissue-derived cells [73] for patients with dry AMD and GA in a pilot phase 1/2a trial (Fig. 2) [66]. To achieve subretinal delivery, the scleral incision was created more posteriorly 8–11 mm behind the

Fig. 1 Suprachoroidal tunneled catheter used for posterior segment gene delivery. The flexible catheter [9] is introduced into the suprachoroidal space [7] via a sclerotomy [8] and is guided into the posterior submacular or peripapillary region using a fiber-optic light source that illuminates the tip. Figure used with permission, originally published in Am J Ophthalmol, Vol 142, Olsen et al., Cannulation of the Suprachoroidal Space: A Novel Drug Delivery Methodology to the Posterior Segment, Pg 777–787. Copyright Elsevier (2006)

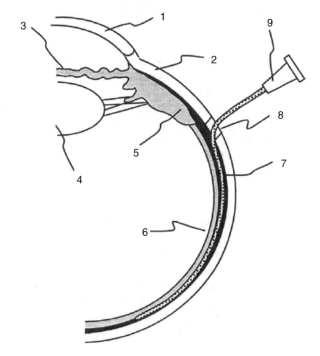

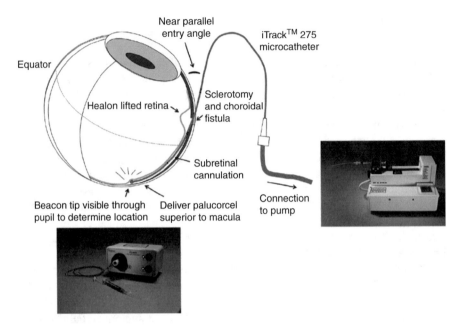

Fig. 2 The suprachoroidal-to-subretinal tunneled microcatheter is introduced via a sclerotomy and choroidotomy into the subretinal space where it is tunneled posteriorly to deliver subretinal cell therapy. An initial subretinal bleb is formed using viscoelastic to elevate the retina over the site where the catheter enters. Figure used with permission, originally published in Am J Ophthalmol, Vol 179, Ho et al., Experience With a Subretinal Cell-based Therapy in Patients With Geographic Atrophy Secondary to Age-related Macular Degeneration, Pg 67–80. Copyright Elsevier (2017)

limbus. A microcannula was passed through both the sclerotomy and choroid, and subretinal sodium hyaluronate viscoelastic was injected to create a subretinal bleb. Then, the microcatheter was introduced through the choroidotomy into the subretinal space and tunnelled under the retina until the tip was adjacent to the area of GA. Subretinal Palucorcel therapy was well tolerated without a significant immune response when given through this method [66], although the technique was associated with retinal perforation. A modified version of the device, iTrack 400 (iScience Interventional Corporation, Menlo Park, California, USA), was subsequently developed and tested for suprachoroidal-only delivery in a clinical trial [74]. However, the goal of the trial was the sub macular suprachoroidal deposition of triamcinolone and bevacizumab, an anti-VEGF monoclonal antibody, rather than gene delivery. Using this method, drugs could be successfully delivered without significant adverse events.

The next suprachoroidal microcatheter iteration utilised a novel, specially designed microcatheter designed for microinjection into the subretinal space. Similar to prior designs, this approach utilised a flexible catheter which could be atraumatically passed through the SCS but featured several advancements (Fig. 3). The catheter tip housed an advanceable microneedle which could be extended with a micro-adjustment knob. Once the catheter was tunnelled posteriorly to the desired

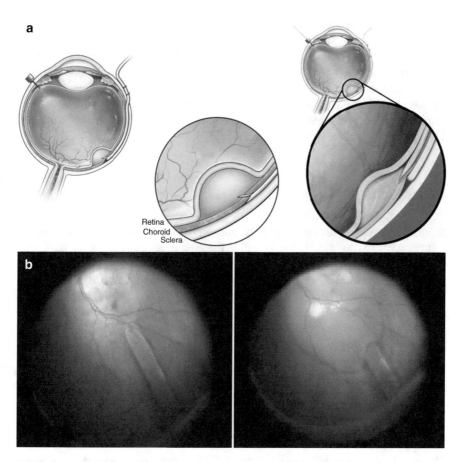

Fig. 3 Suprachoroidal tunneled microcatheter for subretinal injection using the Orbit Subretinal Delivery System (**a**). A microneedle is extended from the cannula tip under direct surgeon visualisation and control to create a subretinal bleb in the posterior pole for delivery of potential cell or gene therapies to the subretinal space without creating a retinotomy (**b**)

location, the operator could advance the needle through the choroid and RPE to inject into the subretinal space under direct visualisation by the operating room microscope. A third-arm positioning tool was used to fix the device onto an armrest in the operating field. This stabilised the alignment of the catheter and reduced the need for free holding of the catheter. A balanced salt solution (BSS) entry bleb was first created before the delivery of cells. The fluid path for BSS is separate from cell delivery, so the procedure could be aborted if retinal penetration occurred without inadvertent injection of cells. The device was successfully tested in minipigs and could reliably deliver subretinal BSS and cells [43]. This led to a phase 1/2a study of Palucorcel injected into the subretinal space using the new device in patients with dry AMD and GA [42]. The study found that the full dose treatment could be successfully delivered in 86% of participants. There were no procedure-related adverse events such as retinal detachment, significant choroidal haemorrhage, retinal perforation, or unintended cell egress. The Orbit Subretinal Delivery System (Orbit SDS, Orbit Biomedical, a subsidiary of Gyroscope Therapeutics, London, United Kingdom) is now being utilised in an investigational hESC-derived human RPE cell suspension therapy trial for atrophic AMD (Lineage Cell Therapeutics, Carlsbad, California, USA) [75]. The next generation of the Orbit SDS is intended to be employed in an investigational gene therapy trial for atrophic AMD (Gyroscope Therapeutics, London, United Kingdom) [36].

Conclusion

Surgical approaches for suprachoroidal and suprachoroidal-to-subretinal gene and cell therapy delivery continue to be refined as new treatment modalities are developed.The safety, efficacy and durability of emerging therapies will also need to be validated in the context of their delivery method. More research is warranted to improve technique-related safety, ease of use, and reproducibility of the current generation methodologies. The potential advantages of therapeutic delivery via the SCS warrant further research and development in the field.

References

1. Garafalo AV, Cideciyan AV, Héon E, et al. Progress in treating inherited retinal diseases: early subretinal gene therapy clinical trials and candidates for future initiatives. Prog Retin Eye Res. 2019;100827
2. Takahashi VKL, Takiuti JT, Jauregui R, Tsang SH. Gene therapy in inherited retinal degenerative diseases, a review. Ophthalmic Genet. 2018;39:560–8.
3. Lee JH, Wang J-H, Chen J, et al. Gene therapy for visual loss: opportunities and concerns. Prog Retin Eye Res. 2019;68:31–53.
4. Stout JT, Francis PJ. Surgical approaches to gene and stem cell therapy for retinal disease. Hum Gene Ther. 2011;22:531–5.
5. Cukras C, Wiley HE, Jeffrey BG, et al. Retinal AAV8-RS1 gene therapy for X-linked retinoschisis: initial findings from a phase I/IIa trial by intravitreal delivery. Mol Ther. 2018;26:2282–94.
6. Ratican SE, Osborne A, Martin KR. Progress in gene therapy to prevent retinal ganglion cell loss in Glaucoma and Leber's hereditary optic neuropathy. Neural Plast 2018;2018. https://www.ncbi.nlm.nih.gov/pmc/articles/PMC5954906/. Accessed 3 May 2020.
7. Dalkara D, Kolstad KD, Caporale N, et al. Inner limiting membrane barriers to AAV-mediated retinal transduction from the vitreous. Mol Ther. 2009;17:2096–102.
8. Campbell JP, McFarland TJ, Stout JT. Ocular gene therapy. Dev Ophthalmol. 2016;55:317–21.
9. Singh R, Cuzzani O, Binette F, et al. Pluripotent stem cells for retinal tissue engineering: current status and future prospects. Stem Cell Rev Rep. 2018;14:463–83.
10. Singh MS, Park SS, Albini TA, et al. Retinal stem cell transplantation: balancing safety and potential. Prog Retin Eye Res. 2020;75:100779.
11. Gu SM, Thompson DA, Srikumari CR, et al. Mutations in RPE65 cause autosomal recessive childhood-onset severe retinal dystrophy. Nat Genet. 1997;17:194–7.

12. Russell S, Bennett J, Wellman JA, et al. Efficacy and safety of voretigene neparvovec (AAV2-hRPE65v2) in patients with RPE65-mediated inherited retinal dystrophy: a randomised, controlled, open-label, phase 3 trial. Lancet. 2017;390:849–60.
13. Bainbridge JWB, Smith AJ, Barker SS, et al. Effect of gene therapy on visual function in Leber's congenital amaurosis. N Engl J Med. 2008;358:2231–9.
14. Edwards TL, Jolly JK, Groppe M, et al. Visual acuity after retinal gene therapy for choroideremia. N Engl J Med. 2016;374:1996–8.
15. MacLaren RE, Groppe M, Barnard AR, et al. Retinal gene therapy in patients with choroideremia: initial findings from a phase 1/2 clinical trial. Lancet. 2014;383:1129–37.
16. Sankila EM, Tolvanen R, van den Hurk JA, et al. Aberrant splicing of the CHM gene is a significant cause of choroideremia. Nat Genet. 1992;1:109–13.
17. Guy J, Feuer WJ, Davis JL, et al. Gene therapy for Leber hereditary optic neuropathy. Ophthalmology. 2017;124:1621–34.
18. Wan X, Pei H, Zhao M, et al. Efficacy and safety of rAAV2-ND4 treatment for Leber's hereditary optic neuropathy. Sci Rep. 2016;6:21587.
19. Cehajic-Kapetanovic J, Xue K, Martinez-Fernandez de la Camara C, et al. Initial results from a first-in-human gene therapy trial on X-linked retinitis pigmentosa caused by mutations in RPGR. Nat Med. 2020;26:354–9.
20. Kahle NA, Peters T, Zobor D, et al. Development of methodology and study protocol: safety and efficacy of a single subretinal injection of rAAV.hCNGA3 in patients with CNGA3-linked achromatopsia investigated in an exploratory dose-escalation trial. Hum Gene Ther Clin Dev. 2018;29:121–31.
21. Fischer MD, Michalakis S, Wilhelm B, et al. Safety and vision outcomes of subretinal gene therapy targeting cone photoreceptors in achromatopsia: a nonrandomized controlled trial. JAMA Ophthalmol. 2020;138(6):643–51.
22. Rodrigues GA, Shalaev E, Karami TK, et al. Pharmaceutical development of AAV-based gene therapy products for the eye. Pharm Res. 2019;36:29.
23. Ramlogan-Steel CA, Murali A, Andrzejewski S, et al. Gene therapy and the adeno-associated virus in the treatment of genetic and acquired ophthalmic diseases in humans: trials, future directions and safety considerations. Clin Exp Ophthalmol. 2019;47:521–36.
24. Balaggan KS, Ali RR. Ocular gene delivery using lentiviral vectors. Gene Ther. 2012;19:145–53.
25. Cavalieri V, Baiamonte E, Lo IM. Non-primate lentiviral vectors and their applications in gene therapy for ocular disorders. Viruses. 2018;10
26. Cremers FPM, Lee W, Collin RWJ, Allikmets R. Clinical spectrum, genetic complexity and therapeutic approaches for retinal disease caused by ABCA4 mutations. Prog Retin Eye Res. 2020;100861
27. Parker MA, Choi D, Erker LR, et al. Test-retest variability of functional and structural parameters in patients with Stargardt disease participating in the SAR422459 gene therapy trial. Transl Vis Sci Technol. 2016;5:10.
28. Trapani I, Puppo A, Auricchio A. Vector platforms for gene therapy of inherited retinopathies. Prog Retin Eye Res. 2014;43:108–28.
29. Heier JS, Kherani S, Desai S, et al. Intravitreous injection of AAV2-sFLT01 in patients with advanced neovascular age-related macular degeneration: a phase 1, open-label trial. Lancet. 2017;390:50–61.
30. Constable IJ, Pierce CM, Lai C-M, et al. Phase 2a randomized clinical trial: safety and post hoc analysis of subretinal rAAV.sFLT-1 for wet age-related macular degeneration. EBioMedicine. 2016;14:168–75.
31. Campochiaro PA, Lauer AK, Sohn EH, et al. Lentiviral vector gene transfer of endostatin/angiostatin for macular degeneration (GEM) study. Hum Gene Ther. 2017;28:99–111.
32. Hemera Biosciences. Treatment of advanced dry age related macular degeneration with AAVCAGsCD59. ClinicalTrials.gov. https://clinicaltrials.gov/ct2/show/NCT03144999. Accessed 9 May 2020.

33. Brown DM, Michels M, Kaiser PK, et al. Ranibizumab versus verteporfin photodynamic therapy for neovascular age-related macular degeneration: Two-year results of the ANCHOR study. Ophthalmology. 2009;116:57–65.e5.
34. Rosenfeld PJ, Brown DM, Heier JS, et al. Ranibizumab for neovascular age-related macular degeneration. N Engl J Med. 2006;355:1419–31.
35. Heier JS, Brown DM, Chong V, et al. Intravitreal aflibercept (VEGF trap-eye) in wet age-related macular degeneration. Ophthalmology. 2012;119:2537–48.
36. Gyroscope Therapeutics. First in human study to evaluate the safety and efficacy of gt005 administered in subjects with dry AMD. ClinicalTrials.gov. https://clinicaltrials.gov/ct2/show/NCT03846193. Accessed 9 May 2020.
37. da Cruz L, Fynes K, Georgiadis O, et al. Phase 1 clinical study of an embryonic stem cell-derived retinal pigment epithelium patch in age-related macular degeneration. Nat Biotechnol. 2018;36:328–37.
38. Kashani AH, Uang J, Mert M, et al. Surgical method for implantation of a biosynthetic retinal pigment epithelium monolayer for geographic atrophy: experience from a phase 1/2a study. Ophthalmol Retina. 2020;4:264–73.
39. Kashani AH, Lebkowski JS, Rahhal FM, et al. A bioengineered retinal pigment epithelial monolayer for advanced, dry age-related macular degeneration. Sci Transl Med. 2018;10
40. Kashani AH, Martynova A, Koss M, et al. Subretinal implantation of a human embryonic stem cell-derived retinal pigment epithelium monolayer in a porcine model. Adv Exp Med Biol. 2019;1185:569–74.
41. Sharma R, Khristov V, Rising A, et al. Clinical-grade stem cell–derived retinal pigment epithelium patch rescues retinal degeneration in rodents and pigs. Sci Transl Med 2019;11. https://stm.sciencemag.org/content/11/475/eaat5580. Accessed 11 May 2020
42. Heier JS, Ho AC, Samuel MA, et al. Safety and efficacy of subretinally administered palucorcel for geographic atrophy of age-related macular degeneration. Ophthalmol Retina. 2020;4:384–93.
43. de Smet MD, Lynch JL, Dejneka NS, et al. A subretinal cell delivery method via suprachoroidal access in minipigs: safety and surgical outcomes. Invest Ophthalmol Vis Sci. 2018;59:311.
44. Ochakovski GA, Bartz-Schmidt KU, Fischer MD. Retinal gene therapy: surgical vector delivery in the translation to clinical trials. Front Neurosci. 2017;11. https://www.frontiersin.org/articles/10.3389/fnins.2017.00174/full. Accessed 3 May 2020
45. Feuer WJ, Schiffman JC, Davis JL, et al. Gene therapy for Leber hereditary optic neuropathy: initial results. Ophthalmology. 2016;123:558–70.
46. Yang S, Ma S-Q, Wan X, et al. Long-term outcomes of gene therapy for the treatment of Leber's hereditary optic neuropathy. EBioMedicine. 2016;10:258–68.
47. Zhang Y, Tian Z, Yuan J, et al. The progress of gene therapy for Leber's optic hereditary neuropathy. Curr Gene Ther. 2018;17:320–6.
48. Kotterman MA, Yin L, Strazzeri JM, et al. Antibody neutralisation poses a barrier to intravitreal adeno-associated viral vector gene delivery to non-human primates. Gene Ther. 2015;22:116–26.
49. Reichel FF, Peters T, Wilhelm B, et al. Humoral immune response after intravitreal but not after subretinal AAV8 in primates and patients. Invest Ophthalmol Vis Sci. 2018;59:1910–5.
50. Timmers AM, Newmark JA, Turunen HT, et al. Ocular inflammatory response to intravitreal injection of adeno-associated virus vector: relative contribution of genome and capsid. Hum Gene Ther. 2019;31:80–9.
51. Grishanin R, Vuillemenot B, Sharma P, et al. Preclinical evaluation of ADVM-022, a novel gene therapy approach to treating wet age-related macular degeneration. Mol Ther. 2019;27:118–29.
52. Xue K, Groppe M, Salvetti AP, MacLaren RE. Technique of retinal gene therapy: delivery of viral vector into the subretinal space. Eye (Lond). 2017;31:1308–16.
53. Hauswirth WW, Aleman TS, Kaushal S, et al. Treatment of leber congenital amaurosis due to RPE65 mutations by ocular subretinal injection of adeno-associated virus gene vector: short-term results of a phase I trial. Hum Gene Ther. 2008;19:979–90.

54. Testa F, Maguire AM, Rossi S, et al. Three-year follow-up after unilateral subretinal delivery of adeno-associated virus in patients with Leber congenital Amaurosis type 2. Ophthalmology. 2013;120:1283–91.
55. Kansara V, Muya L, Wan C, Ciulla TA. Suprachoroidal delivery of viral and nonviral gene therapy for retinal diseases. J Ocular Pharmacol Therap. 2020;36(6):384–92.
56. Spencer R, Fisher S, Lewis GP, Malone T. Epiretinal membrane in a subject after transvitreal delivery of palucorcel (CNTO 2476). Clin Ophthalmol. 2017;11:1797–803.
57. Patel SR, Berezovsky DE, McCarey BE, et al. Targeted administration into the suprachoroidal space using a microneedle for drug delivery to the posterior segment of the eye. Invest Ophthalmol Vis Sci. 2012;53:4433–41.
58. Wang M, Liu W, Lu Q, et al. Pharmacokinetic comparison of ketorolac after intracameral, intravitreal, and suprachoroidal administration in rabbits. Retina (Philadelphia, Pa). 2012;32:2158–64.
59. Kim YC, Edelhauser HF, Prausnitz MR. Targeted delivery of antiglaucoma drugs to the supraciliary space using microneedles. Invest Ophthalmol Vis Sci. 2014;55:7387–97.
60. Patel SR, Lin ASP, Edelhauser HF, Prausnitz MR. Suprachoroidal drug delivery to the back of the eye using hollow microneedles. Pharm Res. 2011;28:166–76.
61. Hackett SF, Fu J, Kim YC, et al. Sustained delivery of acriflavine from the suprachoroidal space provides long term suppression of choroidal neovascularisation. Biomaterials. 2020;243:119935.
62. Yeh S, Khurana RN, Shah M, et al. Efficacy and safety of suprachoroidal CLS-TA for macular edema secondary to noninfectious uveitis. Ophthalmology. 2020;S0161642020300117
63. Campochiaro PA, Wykoff CC, Brown DM, et al. Suprachoroidal triamcinolone Acetonide for retinal vein occlusion: results of the tanzanite study. Ophthalmol Retina. 2018;2:320–8.
64. Goldstein DA, Do D, Noronha G, et al. Suprachoroidal corticosteroid administration: a novel route for local treatment of noninfectious uveitis. Transl Vis Sci Technol. 2016;5:14.
65. Tyagi P, Barros M, Stansbury JW, Kompella UB. Light-activated, in situ forming gel for sustained suprachoroidal delivery of bevacizumab. Mol Pharm. 2013;10:2858–67.
66. Ho AC, Chang TS, Samuel M, et al. Experience with a subretinal cell-based therapy in patients with geographic atrophy secondary to age-related macular degeneration. Am J Ophthalmol. 2017;179:67–80.
67. Ding K, Shen J, Hafiz Z, et al. AAV8-vectored suprachoroidal gene transfer produces widespread ocular transgene expression. J Clin Investig. 2019;129:4901–11.
68. Yiu G, Chung SH, Mollhoff IN, et al. Suprachoroidal and subretinal injections of AAV using transscleral microneedles for retinal gene delivery in nonhuman primates. Mol Ther. 2020;16:179–91.
69. Hartman RR, Kompella UB. Intravitreal, subretinal, and suprachoroidal injections: evolution of microneedles for drug delivery. J Ocul Pharmacol Ther. 2018;34:141–53.
70. Sarin H. Physiologic upper limits of pore size of different blood capillary types and another perspective on the dual pore theory of microvascular permeability. J Angiogenes Res. 2010;2:14.
71. Olsen TW, Feng X, Wabner K, et al. Cannulation of the suprachoroidal space: a novel drug delivery methodology to the posterior segment. Am J Ophthalmol. 2006;142:777–87.
72. Peden MC, Min J, Meyers C, et al. Ab-externo AAV-mediated gene delivery to the suprachoroidal space using a 250 micron flexible microcatheter Qiu J, ed. PLoS One. 2011;6:e17140.
73. Lund RD, Wang S, Lu B, et al. Cells isolated from umbilical cord tissue rescue photoreceptors and visual functions in a rodent model of retinal disease. Stem Cells. 2007;25:602–11.
74. Tetz M, Rizzo S, Augustin AJ. Safety of submacular suprachoroidal drug administration via a microcatheter: retrospective analysis of European treatment results. Ophthalmologica. 2012;227:183–9.
75. Lineage Cell Therapeutics. Safety and efficacy study of OpRegen for treatment of advanced dry-form age-related macular degeneration. ClinicalTrials.gov. https://clinicaltrials.gov/ct2/show/NCT02286089?term=OpRegen&recrs=ab&rank=1. Accessed 11 May 2020.

The Development of a Suprachoroidal Retinal Prosthesis

Penelope J. Allen and Jonathan Yeoh

There is evidence both from human histopathology and animal models of retinal dystrophy that preservation of neuronal elements of the inner retina occurs long after photoreceptors have been lost [1, 2]. The basic theory behind the development of retinal prostheses is that stimulation of these residual neuronal elements, either with electricity or light, can generate a visual percept, also known as a phosphene.

Interestingly, although external electrical stimulation of the eye had been known to produce visual perception as early as the eighteenth century, due to reports by Volta and others, limitations in technology and surgical techniques prevented attempts to implant vision prostheses until the mid-twentieth century. The first known patent and published description of a retinal prosthesis were by G.E. Tassicker in Melbourne in 1956 [3].

A clinically effective retinal prosthesis must evoke localised phosphenes in a retinotopic manner in response to stimulation of each of the retinal electrodes, portray brightness cues over a wide dynamic range and function within safe stimulus limits.

The more recent advances in microsurgery and engineering have enabled numerous groups worldwide to explore different surgical approaches using various devices in an attempt to provide low level electrical stimulation which can safely and reliably produce phosphenes. These surgical approaches are classified according to the position of the device within the eye in relation to the retina.

The device can be placed in the epiretinal position, for example, and the Argus I™ by Second Sight Medical Products was the first iteration of an epiretinal device with

P. J. Allen (✉) · J. Yeoh
Centre for Eye Research Australia, Royal Victorian Eye and Ear Hospital, East Melbourne, VIC, Australia

Department of Surgery (Ophthalmology), The University of Melbourne, Parkville, VIC, Australia
e-mail: pjallen@melbourneretina.com.au

16-electrodes. The second-generation Argus II™, a 60-electrode device received FDA regulatory approval in 2011, however, production of this device has now been discontinued [4]. Several groups have used the subretinal approach, the most notable being Retinal Implant AG from Germany. They have developed two devices, the first-generation Alpha IMS™ and the second-generation Alpha AMS™ [5, 6]. Both have been successful in clinical trials and have been approved through the EU regulatory processes (CE Mark) although commercial production of the Retinal Implant AG subretinal device has also been ceased. More recently Pixium Vision has announced early results of their PRIMA photovoltaic subretinal device implanted in patients with geographic atrophy due to age related macular degeneration [7].

The Japanese retinal prosthesis group, lead until recently by Prof Takashi Fujikado, developed a suprachoroidal intrascleral device placed within a scleral flap [8]. This has been used in a human clinical trial but has not been commercialised.

The path to our Australian retinal prosthesis trials commenced with an invitation by Hugh Taylor to Mark McCombe and the author (P. Allen) to collaborate with Gregg Suaning and Nigel Lovell at the University of New South Wales to develop a suprachoroidal surgical approach for a retinal prosthesis that was being developed in collaboration with a team in South Korea. This initial development work was conducted using a rabbit model.

In 2008 the Australia 2020 summit was held in Canberra, Australia.

The Long term National Health Strategy initiative to develop a bionic eye was funded by the Australian Research Council for the purpose of developing an Australian bionic eye.

Our collaborative group was awarded this funding. Monash Vision Group was the other successful applicant for their work on a cortical prosthesis.

Bionic Vision Australia was a collaboration between the Centre for Eye Research Australia, the Bionics Institute, the University of New South Wales, the University of Melbourne and National ICT Australia Ltd., with additional partners. The plan was to bring the University of New South Wales device to clinical trial and do preliminary development work on the University of Melbourne nanocrystalline diamond epiretinal device. The Centre for Eye Research Australia's involvement was in preclinical work collaborating with the Bionics Institute, clinical work preparing for human trial and finally in running the clinical trial.

It became apparent that the UNSW device was not going to be ready for human implantation. The suprachoroidal approach, however, remained very attractive, particularly due to the simplicity and ease of surgery, but more development work was required. Surgical development had to proceed collaboratively and in parallel with preclinical and clinical development such that a safe and effective device can be produced for testing.

Robert Shepherd's extensive experience with Cochlear implants made him the perfect lead for the preclinical team, and Robyn Guymer's clinical trial experience was essential to prepare for and run a clinical trial. The surgical and engineering teams developed the electrode array, and device and the clinical team refined a database of patients with end stage retinal dystrophies who could potentially be suitable candidates once the device came to the human clinical trial.

The feline model had previously been used for cochlear implant work, and this was chosen as the animal model for the suprachoroidal device due to the similar sizes of the feline and human eye. The extensive library of work relating to the visual cortex in cats also guided and facilitated performing visual psychophysics during the preclinical development of the device. The development of a surgical model required dissections of feline eyes to study with their ocular and orbital anatomy. Ongoing development of modifications to existing surgical techniques in the human eye was made in adjustment to the feline ocular model.

We were guided in the surgical development work by Chris Williams of the Bionics Institute.

The initial surgeries were to demonstrate the proof of concept, that stimulation within the suprachoroidal space (SCS) could produce measurable responses within the visual cortex of the feline animal model. A platinum electrode array was implanted in normally sighted cats, and multiunit activity from the primary visual cortex was recorded in response to varying modes of stimulation. Threshold, the yield of responses, dynamic range and the spread of retinal activation were measured for these varying modes [9].

Multiunit activity in the primary visual cortex was recorded in response to electrical stimulation using various return configurations to determine the most charge efficient stimulation to induce cortical activity within safe charge limits [10].

These studies were also used to develop the form and footprint of the device, which could be slightly modified at a later date for the human device. We were able to demonstrate that the suprachoroidal array could be reliably positioned beneath the area centralis in the feline model, that retinal folding only occurred if the device was inserted too close to the optic nerve and that in no case did the array breach the retina, choroid or sclera [11].

We performed two groups of chronic studies. Firstly, passive studies were performed to demonstrate that the device was conformable and stable in position long term. To demonstrate this, we implanted the devices in normally sighted cats for 3 months. Surgical stability and ocular health were assessed with fundus photography and electroretinography (ERG). At the end of 3 months, the animals were sacrificed, and the eyes collected for histopathology. The imaging and ERG data confirmed that the devices were stable and that retinal function remained normal. The histopathology showed that the retina was intact and there was minimal foreign body response to the device, hence confirming that the device was stable and well tolerated over the 3 month period [12].

The second group of chronic studies involved active stimulation of the implanted suprachoroidal devices for 70–105 days to demonstrate the safety and efficacy of stimulation of the device in the feline suprachoroidal space over this period. In this study, we stimulated the animals at a level above threshold for 24 h per day. Charge balanced, biphasic current pulses were delivered to the platinum electrodes in a monopolar stimulation mode. Retinal integrity and function, as well as the implant's mechanical stability, were assessed monthly using ERG, optical coherence tomography (OCT) and fundus photography.

Weekly measurements of electrode impedances and monthly measurements of electrically evoked visual cortex potentials (eEVCPs) were used to verify that chronic stimuli were above the threshold. At the end of the chronic stimulation period, thresholds were confirmed with multiunit recordings from the visual cortex. Randomised, blinded histological assessments were performed by two pathologists to compare the stimulated and non-stimulated retina and adjacent tissue. We were able to show at the end of the study that chronic suprathreshold electrical stimulation of the retina by a suprachoroidal electrode array using charge balanced stimulus currents evoked a minimal tissue response with no adverse clinical or histological findings. Furthermore, thresholds and electrode impedance remained stable for stimulation durations of up to 15 weeks [13].

As an additional study to aid our plans for a human clinical trial, we also conducted a chronic study to investigate whether our arrays could be safely explanted or replaced in our feline model. This study consisted of 13 animals. One month after implantation arrays were surgically explanted ($n = 6$), replaced ($n = 5$) or left in situ ($n = 2$) undisturbed. The fundus was then assessed using fundus photography and OCT during and at the end of the study. Three months after the initial implantation, the arrays were assessed by measuring responses in the visual cortex to electrical stimulation of the arrays. The retina was further assessed with histology. We were able to show that explantation or replacement was successful in all cases and clinical assessment with fundus photography did not show any additional changes in these cases compared to the animals with the devices left in situ. Early OCT assessment after replacement showed some increase in the electrode to retina distance which settled. Electrode impedances were unchanged during the study, and electrophysiological responses did not differ between the replaced and undisturbed arrays. This gave us confidence that a faulty array could be removed or replaced with no significant damage to the retina [14].

Until this point our work had been conducted in a normal feline model, so we collaborated with Felix Aplin and Erica Fletcher to develop a feline retinal degeneration model to test our suprachoroidal stimulation in. We hypothesised that stimulation thresholds would differ between the eye with induced photoreceptor degeneration and the normal eye but were keen to know the extent of this difference. The results showed that spatial and temporal cortical responses did not differ between the eyes; however, individual electrode thresholds differed and correlated with ganglion cell density. Within the degenerative eyes thresholds also correlated with the degree of retinal gliosis [15].

These studies gave us the confidence to progress to the next level. We had collected and published more preclinical animal data than any of the other bionic eye groups. However, we still needed to determine that the approach would work in live human tissue and that the successful surgical approach that we had developed could be transferred to human patients.

We had informed our Oculoplastic colleagues that we were interested in performing a pilot surgery in a human patient who would be undergoing enucleation. Human research and ethics committee approval from the Royal Victorian Eye and Ear Hospital in anticipation of such a patient had been granted.

We were subsequently contacted by one of our colleagues who was performing a bilateral enucleation on a female patient. This patient had enquired of her surgeon if there was anything she could do for science. She had been no light perception (NPL) vision in both eyes for many years due to end-stage Retinitis Pigmentosa, which had similarly affected her sister and niece. The patient understood and consented to the fact that it would add significant time to her surgery. We, therefore, proceeded with the insertion of a dummy electrode array into the suprachoroidal space in both eyes prior to enucleation. The histology from this pilot study shows the location of the dummy electrode array within the suprachoroidal space (Fig. 1).

Simultaneously, during this time, human cadaver eye studies were also carried out to help us develop specific design features and surgical strategies for the human eye. We have always regarded the exit point of the lead from the eye to be very important, particularly its potential effect on device stability. The device also required a low profile to minimise any erosion into adjacent tissue resulting in device extrusion, and strong enough to resist the breakage. The cadaver studies were vital for developing these essential aspects of the device [16].

We continued our cadaver work in the Anatomy School at the University of Melbourne in collaboration with ENT surgeon Robert Briggs from the Royal Victorian Eye and Ear Hospital. The aim was to finalise the surgical procedure, determine the additional surgical tools required, develop those tools, and determine the theatre's layout and workflow.

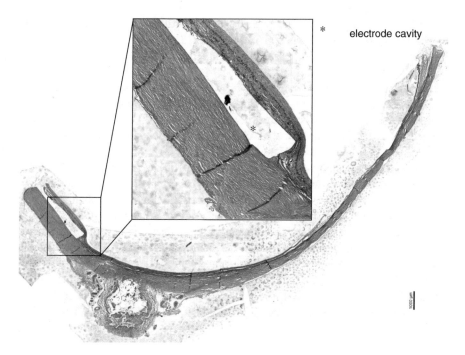

Fig. 1 Histology of human pilot

The fact that the suprachoroidal approach had not been used in humans previously led us to decide to have a percutaneous connector for stimulation. The level and manner of stimulation could be varied. Robert Briggs had experience with this approach for Cochlear implants and collaborated with us to develop strategies for the lead wire and stabilisation of the percutaneous connector. We needed a surgical tool to pass the electrode array forward from the wound created for the percutaneous connector. A specific trocar was designed by Owen Burns from the Bionics Institute for this purpose.

The theatre staff at the Royal Victorian Eye and Ear Hospital (RVEEH) have worked with us to adjust the layout of the operating theatre, plan required standard and new instrumentation for the procedure and its sterilisation.

We wanted to prove prior to submitting an application to the Human Research and Ethics committee that the device was robust and that it could withstand the eye's constant movement without lead breakages. To achieve this, the array underwent bench testing designed to damage it to be confident that surgical insertion would not cause loss of functionality. Also, our colleagues at the Bionics Institute developed a rig to test the leads. Skulls with continuously saccading artificial eyes in which leads were sutured to the eye were used to generate lead fatigue data. Over twenty years of simulated saccadic data were generated with no lead breakages (Fig. 2).

The results were to the satisfaction of clinical and surgical teams before proceeding to the clinical trial application to the Human Research and Ethics Committee at the Royal Victorian Eye and Ear Hospital.

The trial was a proof of concept study, and the patients who entered the study took a leap of faith without knowing the outcome and realising that the percutaneous connector would need to be removed eventually and the device in situ would not be a long term option, even if it worked.

So, what did this trial demonstrate? We were able to complete the surgery with implantation of the first prototype on three patients with no intraoperative complications, and at the end of the surgeries, impedance testing showed that all electrodes in the arrays were fully functional and remained so for the length of the study.

In all three subjects, a combined subretinal and suprachoroidal haemorrhage formed 3–4 days postoperatively, which resolved without any ongoing complications in Patient 1 and Patient 3. In Patient 2, who experienced a larger haemorrhage, an area of preretinal fibrosis remained at the temporal end of the implant following haemorrhage resolution, but this did not affect device efficacy nor caused further complications including retinal detachment. None of the subjects was taking anticoagulant medication during this study. We demonstrated that stimulation in the suprachoroidal space can produce reliable phosphenes and that functional improvement can be achieved with a device that was robust and reliable. The suprachoroidal device was also stable on serial fundus photography and OCT as was the intraorbital component of the device checked with plain X-ray over the duration of the trial [17].

Fig. 2 Lead wire testing, skulls in the cupboard

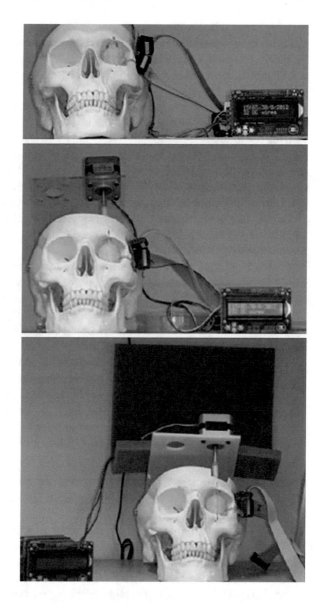

Also, we were able to demonstrate that two of the three patients in the trial were able to navigate with the device, exceeding our expectations for the device's performance.

The collaboration between the Centre for Eye Research Australia team and the investigators from the Bionics Institute continues using the feedback and data from our prototype trial. We are developing the second generation device that is fully implantable and can be used outside the laboratory [18]. The patients from the prototype trial felt that the area of stimulation should be larger in the horizontal plane, so the number of stimulating electrodes was increased to forty four. Due to the increased number of electrodes, the mechanical properties of the electrode array had changed, therefore requiring more development work, preclinical safety and efficacy studies.

We conducted further animal studies, again using the feline model. The implants we placed for up to 20 weeks, and the stability and safety of the device were assessed with the use of fundus photography, OCT, and ERG. The findings confirmed that the second generation device could be inserted safely with good retinal conformability and stability within the suprachoroidal space in the majority of animals. No significant retinal trauma was observed in the study, and only a small number of adverse events occurred, some of which were animal model specific [19].

During this work, driven by David Nayagam, we developed safety limits for stimulation in our animal model, such that we could direct our stimulation strategies for the upcoming human study.

We recruited four patients with advanced retinal dystrophy and visual acuity no better than light perception in all patients for our second human study. All four patients had been unable to navigate themselves for more than ten years. They were implanted with our second generation device in the suprachoroidal space and with an external vision processing unit, which could be used by the patients at home following a period of initial training (Fig. 3).

The clinical trial protocol has been developed from our experience with the initial prototype study. The study aimed to determine the safety and stability of the 44-channel device. As the participants would be able to use the devices outside the laboratory, the study included significant levels of training and rehabilitation, in addition to the assessment of outcome measures such as visual acuity, Orientation and Mobility (O&M) tasks and Activities of Daily Living (ADL). There were 3 phases to the study:

Phase 1: Recovery phase in the early postoperative period after surgery before commencing electrical stimulation. It was expected that this phase would be a maximum of 2 months.

Phase 2: Device fitting phase, where the initial psychophysics testing was completed. This included thresholding and determination of phosphene maps; and training on the use of the camera in the laboratory-based setting.

Phase 3: Take-home phase, where participants could use their device outside the laboratory and without supervision. During this phase, the participants had a 24-h emergency contact number for any concerns and regularly seen at the research site.

The entire study was planned to run for two years. The study's primary endpoint is the safety of the 44ChFI device, as determined by the number of device-related serious adverse events (SAEs). The secondary endpoint is the efficacy of the 44ChFI device, as determined by outcome assessments of visual acuity and functional vision (O&M and ADL).

Fig. 3 Second generation
device/system

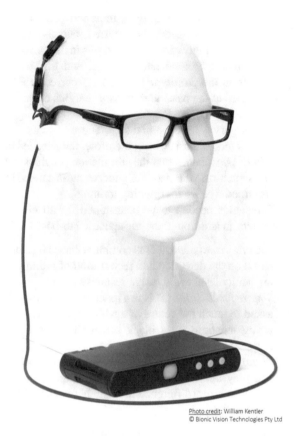

The surgical procedure consists of the implantation of the receiver/stimulator units via an incision superior to the pinna. The electrode array is then tunnelled forward to a lateral canthotomy in preparation for insertion into the suprachoroidal space. A wedge shaped orbitotomy is made below the zygomaticofrontal suture for stabilisation of the lead.

A 180° conjunctival peritomy is made, and the lateral rectus muscle is exposed and disinserted. A full thickness 9 mm scleral cutdown to choroid is made posterior to the insertion of the lateral rectus muscle with the location of the incision determined by preoperative calculations based on the axial length of the eye. The SCS is opened and dissected, and the array is inserted deep into the SCS under the macula. The scleral wound is closed, and the patch for the lead is sutured to the sclera. The position of the device is checked by examination with an indirect ophthalmoscope. After this, the lateral rectus muscle is replaced. The wedge-shaped grommet on the lead is placed within the orbitotomy, and the periosteum closed over this with the help of ENT colleague Robert Briggs.

The soft tissue wounds are closed in layers, and the functional integrity of the device is checked by measuring the impedances to ensure that the surgery has not damaged the device. The surgery took between 204–260 min in our four cases. No intraoperative adverse events occurred, and the patients recovered well after the surgery. Interestingly of the four patients in the current trial, only two developed any postoperative subretinal haemorrhage, and this was very mild compared to the patients from the prototype trial. This occurred in P2 and P4, more marked in P2, both situated at the nasal and inferior margins of the array and cleared rapidly with no sequelae.

The surgery is only the first step. These patients have had no useful visual information for more than 15 years; therefore, they needed to learn to interpret the flashes of light or phosphenes that the stimulation provides during the device fitting phase. After "switch-on" the patients underwent an intensive week of training in the lab and returned weekly for ongoing training.

Thresholds needed to be determined for all electrodes, and a phosphene map generated. In addition, there are specific lab-based tasks:

1. *Grating visual acuity:* This computer-based task determines a visual acuity level based on the detection and recognition of grating optotypes. We record the grating acuity level and average response time.
2. *Square localisation*: This is a touch-screen computer task, where participants are asked to touch the centre of a white square, which is randomly presented in differing locations on a black screen. The response error and response time is measured.
3. *Motion detection*: This computer-based task shows the participant a moving bar, and they are asked to replicate the direction of motion with their hand. The response error (difference in angle between their response and the target bar) is measured.

We also use functional vision tasks to assess the patients:

4. *Table-top search task*: In this task, participants need to locate common household objects on a table, name the object and touch it with their index finger. Accuracy rates and response times are recorded.
5. *The doorway detection task* requires the participant to find and walk to a dark "doorway-shaped" target on a white wall. The start position of the participant and the doorway location are both randomised. Task time and accuracy of the door touch is measured.
6. *Obstacle avoidance task* requires participants to navigate a route which has been seeded with randomly located obstacles. Task time and the number of obstacle collisions are recorded.
7. *The Functional Low Vision Observer Rated Assessment (FLORA)*: This assessment tool, developed as part of the Second Sight Medical Products trials, is used to evaluate the participant's functional vision and mobility in their home environment.

These tasks are used to assess the patient's progress 3 monthly during phase 3 to inform the investigators about the study's secondary endpoints. During the trial, the patient's general and ocular health is monitored regularly. Ocular assessment is made with clinical examination, fundus photography and OCT to ensure any potential adverse events are detected.

Conclusion

The development of a new retinal prosthesis requires a collaborative approach. A solid background of preclinical work has ensured that the progress into a human clinical trial was seamless. The completion of our prototype clinical study of a suprachoroidal retinal prosthesis (NCT01603576) and the commencement and progress of our second generation 44 channel device trial (NCT03406416) demonstrate that we have developed a reproducible surgical procedure with excellent safety profile. The prototype device consistently produced reliable phosphenes within safe charge limits, and two of the three patients in the trial were able to navigate with the second generation 44 channel device. The patients have not completed their two years of the trial, and unfortunately, their outcome measures have been delayed due to the Covid 19 pandemic. However, resumption of the trial is planned, and publication of the lab-based and functional vision tasks results after these final assessments are planned for 2021.

The authors would like to acknowledge the contributions made by the Bionic Eye Research teams from the Centre for Eye Research Australia and the Bionics Institute, without whom this work could not have been completed, and continue productive collaboration between the teams.

References

1. Santos A, Humayun MS, de Juan E Jr, Greenburg RJ, Marsh MJ, Klock IB, Milam AH. Preservation of the inner retina in retinitis pigmentosa. A morphometric analysis. Arch Ophthalmol. 1997;115(4):511–5.
2. Gargini C, Terzibasi E, Mazzoni F, Strettoi E. Retinal organisation in the retinal degeneration 10 (rd10) mutant mouse: a morphological and ERG study. J Comp Neurol. 2007;500(2):222–38.
3. Tassicker GE. Prelininary report of a retinal stimulator. Br J Physiol Optics. 1956;13:2, 102–105.
4. Ahuja AK. Blind subjects implanted with the Argus II retinal prosthesis are able to improve performance in a spatial-motor task. Br J Ophthalmol. 2010;95(4):539–43.
5. Zrenner E. Subretinal electronic chips allow blind patients to read letters and combine them to words. Proc Biol Sci. 2011;278(1711):1489–97.
6. Stingl K, Bartz-Schmidt KU, Besch D, Chee CK, Cottriall CL, Gekeler F, et al. Subretinal visual implant alpha IMS—Clinical trial interim report. Vision Res. 2015;111(Pt B):149–60.
7. Palanker D, Le Mer Y, Mohand-Said S, Muqit M, Sahel JA. Photovoltaic restoration of central vision in atrophic age-related macular degeneration. Ophthalmology. 2020;27(8):1097–104.
8. Fujikado T. Evaluation of phosphenes elicited by extraocular stimulation in normals and by suprachorodal-transretinal stimulation in patients with retinitis pigmentosa. Graefes Arch Clin Exp Ophthalmol. 2007;245(10):1411–9.

9. Shivdasani MN, Fallon JB, Luu CD, Cicione R, Allen PJ, Morley JW, Williams CE. Visual cortex responses to single- and simultaneous multiple-electrode stimulation of the retina: implications for retinal prostheses. Invest Ophth Vis Sci. 2012;53(10):6291–63.
10. Cicione R, Shivdasani MN, Fallon JB, Luu CD, Allen PJ, Rathbone GD, Shepherd RK, Williams CE. Visual cortex responses to suprachoroidal electrical stimulation of the retina: effects of electrode return configuration. J Neural Eng. 2012;9(3)
11. Villalobos J, Allen PJ, McCombe MF, Ulaganathan M, Zamir E, Ng DC, Shepherd RK, Williams CE. Development of a surgical approach for a wide-view suprachoroidal retinal prosthesis: evaluation of implantation trauma. Graef Arch Clin Exp. 2012;250(3):399–407.
12. Villalobos J, Nayagam DAX, Allen PJ, McKelvie P, Luu CD, Ayton LN, Freemantle AL, McPhedran M, Basa M, McGowan CC, et al. A wide-field suprachoroidal retinal prosthesis is stable and well tolerated following chronic implantation. Invest Ophthal Vis Sci. 2013;54(5):3751–62.
13. Nayagam DAX, Williams RA, Allen PJ, Shivdasani MN, Luu CD, Salinas-LaRosa CM, et al. Chronic electrical stimulation with a suprachoroidal retinal prosthesis: a preclinical safety and efficacy study. PLoS One. 2014;9(5)
14. Leung RT, Nayagam DAX, Williams RA, Allen PJ, Salinas-La Rosa CM, Luu CD, et al. Safety and efficacy of explanting or replacing suprachoroidal electrode arrays in a feline model. Clin Exp Ophthalmol. 2015;43(3):247–58.
15. Aplin FP, Fletcher EL, Luu CD, Vessey KA, Allen PJ, Guymer RH, et al. Stimulation of a suprachoroidal retinal prosthesis drives cortical responses in a feline model of retinal degeneration. Invest Ophthalmol Vis Sci. 2016;57(13):5216–29.
16. Saunders AL, Williams CE, Heriot W, Briggs R, Yeoh J, Nayagam DA, et al. Development of a surgical procedure for implantation of a prototype suprachoroidal retinal prosthesis. Clin Exp Ophthalmol. 2014;42(7):665–74.
17. Ayton LN, Blamey PJ, Guymer RH, Luu CD, Nayagam DAX, Sinclair NC, et al. First-in-human trial of a novel suprachoroidal retinal prosthesis. PLoS One. 2014;9(12):1–26.
18. Petoe M, McCarthy C, Shivdasani M, Sinclair N, Scott A, Ayton L, et al. Determining the contribution of retinotopic discrimination to localisation performance with a suprachoroidal retinal prosthesis. Invest Ophthalmol Vis Sci. 2017;58(7):3231.
19. Abbott CJ, Nayagam DAX, Luu CD, Epp SB, Williams RA, Salinas-LaRosa CM, et al. Safety studies for a 44-channel suprachoroidal retinal prosthesis: a chronic passive study. Invest Ophthalmol Vis Sci. 2018;59(3):1410–24.

Printed in the United States
by Baker & Taylor Publisher Services